Women's Health Movements

Women's Health Movements

A Global Force for Change

Meredeth Turshen

First published in 2007 by
PALGRAVE MACMILLAN™
175 Fifth Avenue, New York, N.Y. 10010 and
Houndmills, Basingstoke, Hampshire, England RG21 6XS
Companies and representatives throughout the world.

PALGRAVE MACMILLAN is the global academic imprint of the Palgrave Macmillan division of St. Martin's Press, LLC and of Palgrave Macmillan Ltd. Macmillan® is a registered trademark in the United States, United Kingdom and other countries. Palgrave is a registered trademark in the European Union and other countries.

ISBN 978-1-4039-7898-1   ISBN 978-0-230-60712-5 (eBook)
DOI 10.1057/9780230607125

Library of Congress Cataloging-in-Publication Data

Turshen, Meredeth
     Women's health movements : a global force for change / Meredeth Turshen.
          p. cm.
     Includes bibliographical references and index.

     1. Women—Health and hygiene—Social aspects. 2. Women—International cooperation. 3. Women—Social conditions.
     4. Feminism—Health aspects. 5. Social movements. 6. Women's rights.
     I. Title.

RA564.85.T87 2007
362.1082—dc22   2007005037

A catalogue record for this book is available from the British Library.

Design by Newgen Imaging Systems (P) Ltd., Chennai, India.

Cover art, *Moroccan women* by Meredeth Turshen

First edition: October 2007

10 9 8 7 6 5 4 3 2 1

Transferred to digital printing in 2009.

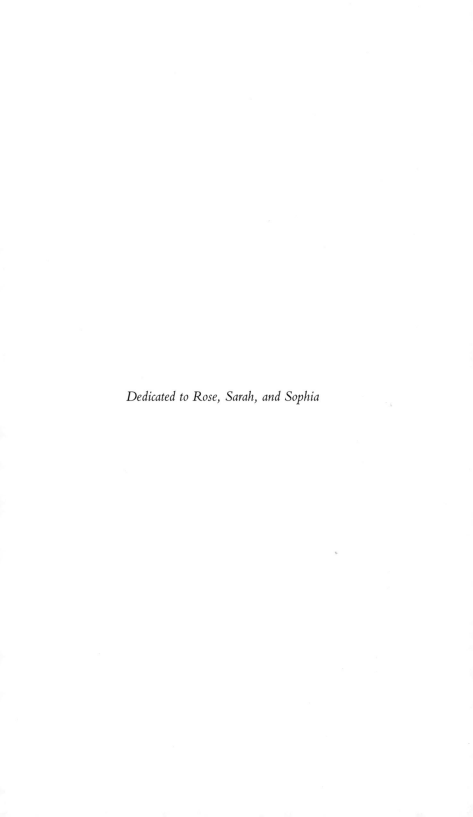

Dedicated to Rose, Sarah, and Sophia

CONTENTS

LIST OF TABLES

ACKNOWLEDGMENTS

My grateful thanks to Asma Abdel Halim for her friendship and inspiration; Charlotte Bunch, from whom I learned so much about women's movements and women's rights; Nonceba Lubanga, Quarraisha Abdool Karim, and Barbara Klugman who introduced me to the politics of women's health in South Africa; Codou Bop for her leadership in Senegal; Kathleen Spivack and Mary Meader Mokler who encouraged me with that old Oberlin spirit; Annie Thébaud-Mony, my coconspirator; Malika Ladjali, merci beaucoup; students in my courses on Contemporary Issues in Women's Health at Rutgers University; Sejal Dave for her enthusiastic research assistance, hard work, and resourcefulness; Blue Mountain Center and Vermont Studio Center, which provided nature and nurture, the essential ingredients of all creative work; Cecile and Jerry Shore for their enduring support; and Google, without which it would not have been possible to do the research for this book. Thanks, too, to Judy Norsigian, Norma Swenson, and the other members of the original Boston Women's Health Book Collective for their inspiring work; and I wish I could thank the late Irv Zola for giving me the key to "universalism."

To my editors at Palgrave Macmillan, Gabriella Georgiades, Joanna Mericle, and to Newgen's Maran Elancheran (the best of "which hunters"), a big thank you.

This book clearly owes its deepest debts to women the world over who sacrificed so much to improve women's health and health care.

CHAPTER ONE

Women Organizing: Activism Worldwide

Prologue: A Personal/Political Statement

For nearly a decade I have wanted, with a growing sense of urgency, to write something that would show what the women's health movement has meant to the women of my generation, the generation of girls who came of age in the 1950s and 60s, became activists in the causes of others, then turned to help one another and, finally, to help ourselves. We grew up in New York, the Casbah of Algiers, the bantustans of South Africa, dusty Khartoum, provincial France, the North of England, and Old Delhi. Each of us carries, on her body and in her mind, a site of humiliation, a scar of betrayed trust, a flashback to an indignity as vivid today as when inflicted. We shared those humiliations, examined each other's scars, and raged at the indignities. I am still enraged.

This book is about sexuality, violence, reproduction, disability—women's health issues and the movements that women created to confront them. The issues are international and larger than medical care: women oppose conflict and war, the debt crisis, shortages of water, food, and work. The most oppressed women urge action on the most basic issues: eliminate poverty, unemployment, poor housing, deteriorating environments, and punishing welfare, immigration, and policing programs. They entreat their governments to provide any kind of medical care and public health services for their neglected communities.

Women's health movements deprecate the ways that society uses medical care to control women's sexuality. We condemn the medical profession for so long ignoring the signs of domestic violence. We reject the condescending, paternalistic, judgmental, uninformative, and infantilizing treatment that is routine in visits to gynecologists and obstetricians. We abhor health workers' participation in unnecessary, unwanted, and punitive sterilizations; unethical clinical trials of contraceptive drugs and devices; and denial of access to abortion. Women are appalled by doctors' willingness to replace healthy breasts with health-damaging implants, to mutilate girls' genitals, and to condone torture.

Talking to one another and analyzing our experiences, women uncovered the gender stereotypes that dictate the different medical care that women, lesbians and gay men, and people of color receive. By paying attention to the ways advertising and the media manipulate women, we exposed the malevolent and invidious practices of pharmaceutical companies—the substitution of pricey infant formula for free breast milk; the marketing of carcinogenic hormones at menopause, playing upon women's fear of growing old; and the invention of new conditions for which the industry also creates a profitable treatment—vaginal odors, premenstrual syndrome, generalized anxiety disorder.

In the past four decades, women's health movements have made dramatic changes in health care in the United States. Women pressed for and won legal contraception and abortion. We pushed for more methods of birth control, and we continue to insist that contraception and abortion reach more women of all ages, married or not, whatever their race, income, and education. We sued manufacturers of dangerous drugs and contraceptive devices. By insisting on fully informed consent, we curbed abuse of sterilization, widely performed on the mentally retarded and poor, black, Latina, and Native American women. We tried to reform unethical research procedures and clinical trials of new drugs both at home and abroad (we are still working on it). We changed obstetric care, demanding better access and higher quality care for all women including the poor and women of color. We won better control of birthing technology; we insisted on justification of Caesarian sections; and we questioned the uncontrolled numbers of hysterectomies. We changed doctor/patient relations in routine gynecological examinations, insisting on initial introductions when fully clothed and on explanations of each test and procedure performed. We changed hospital practice to allow partners in the delivery room and to let newborn babies sleep in mothers' rooms to encourage bonding and breastfeeding. We reinstated midwifery and home birth alternatives, noting that midwifery is woman centered whereas obstetrics is baby centered. We forced attention to infertility (now, alas, big business—these things turn on us sometimes). We forced attention to menopause, breaking a taboo. We demanded an alternative to radical mastectomy, the standard treatment of breast cancer for more than 60 years. We pushed for attention to research on women's health and won it in the Women's Health Initiative. We demanded equal medical education for women and got it: in 1965 only 7 percent of physicians were women; today women make up half of the entering class in medical schools. We helped nurses unionize, improve their relations with doctors, fight job discrimination, and get the pay and respect they deserve. We urged recognition of the hidden, informal health care women provide at home, especially to elderly parents. Women lawyers worked for legal reforms and consumer protections; together with the battered women's movement they reformed laws on domestic violence and treatment of rape victims. We created shelters for battered women and rape-crisis hot lines. And we are still working to change attitudes to gender—to lesbians, transsexuals, women athletes, single mothers, obese women, celibate women, immigrant women (have I left someone out?).

Of all our contributions, I think the most enduring are new models of health education based on the demystification of medicine and science. We learned from the Berkeley Free Speech Movement to Question Authority. We drew on the self-help health movement to teach cervical self-examination. From self-help and from traditions of adult education, we turned ourselves into lay practitioners to perform abortions before they were legal and to provide women's health care in all-women clinics. We used consciousness-raising groups, study groups, and peer education techniques to learn about our bodies, to raise our self-esteem, and to discover that yes, the personal is political. We used our powers as consumers to influence the marketplace; we learned to validate experiential knowledge and use it in documenting our claims for change; and we became popular epidemiologists, studying disease patterns in our communities and drawing attention to clusters of unexplained deaths and demanding investigations. We learned to use new technologies like the internet, and we institutionalized our achievements through Web sites, publications, new laws, and transformed facilities. And by paying attention to the need to put our ideas into the mainstream of medical and public health practice, we tried to ensure that the changes would endure.

There were also failures. We failed to take the profit motive out of medical practice, despite our popular, oft-repeated slogan, "Health for People, Not for Profit." If anything, the situation has deteriorated, as the U.S. model of private, for-profit medical care spreads throughout the world. We won reforms of women's health care but we lost the war for universal access to health services. For every victory over the pharmaceutical industry, there were reversals and new dangers. Most of our early victories came after the damage was done—after doctors had prescribed the sedative thalidomide to pregnant women, robbing thousands of babies of their arms and legs, after the Robbins intrauterine contraceptive device had left thousands of women sterile, after silicone breast implants had damaged the health of thousands of women. With evidence of the dangers of marketing products that the industry had not tested adequately, we won safeguards; but with the AIDS epidemic, demands for early marketing of drugs to treat immune deficiency loosened many of those restrictions.

Although we celebrate many successes in the U.S. women's health movement, the improvements are not distributed evenly. Women of color are asking what it would take for them to get access to woman-friendly, high quality services. In the global South—the poor nations of Africa, Asia, and Latin America—women wonder what it would take to replicate the successes of women's health movements in the North. They confront health issues that are the same and different, and obstacles to better health care that are the same and different, always with fewer resources than are available in the North. Women of color in the United States say they have more in common with women in the global South than with middle and upper class white women in their own country. The U.S. Women of Color Delegation to the International Conference on Population and Development held in Cairo in 1994 said,

> We wanted to bring attention to the similarities between the Southern conditions of women in this Northern country [the United States] and women in the Southern countries and to urge our government to act decisively in addressing and rectifying unjust policies and power imbalances within our society and worldwide. (Quoted in Morgen 2002, 68)

The same health issues—sexuality, violence, reproduction, and disability—are intensified by legacies of conquest and colonialism, by ongoing civil conflicts, new forms of global capitalism and religious fundamentalism, by the imperialism of one superpower, and the loss of an alternative vision, as socialism is discredited everywhere and feminism cannot even be named.

Progress in the South is uneven. For the 16th International Day of Action for Women's Health in 2003, a coalition supported by the People's Health Movement made up of women's groups from Cameroon, Chile, India, Philippines, Uganda, the United States, and Yugoslavia campaigned under the banner, "Health for all—health for women!" The coalition called on governments to take responsibility for women's health, to provide primary health care, and to respect women's reproductive and sexual rights. But in the years since the World Health Organization declared "Health for All by the Year 2000," personal income has dropped dramatically in many poor countries. Never a dollar a day—the international definition of poverty—in the poorest African and Asian countries, it is now 61 cents a day in Rwanda, 60 cents in Bangladesh, 43 cents in Sierra Leone, and 27 cents in Congo. One statistic sums up the exploitation of Africans: according to the World Bank (1993) the median age at death in the United States and Europe is 75 years; in Africa it is under 5 years.

In the past 25 years, the G-7 wealthiest nations in the world have used international financial institutions—the World Bank, the International Monetary Fund, and the World Trade Organization—to impose conditions on loans and aid. Nations no longer control national public policy: to qualify for assistance they must follow the neoliberal economic program, cutting government services, eliminating subsidies on food and fuel, devaluing their currency (which raises the prices of imported pharmaceuticals even higher), and privatizing, well, just about everything in sight. Of most concern to women are the privatization of water, health services, and education.

These loan conditions masquerade as economic reforms. Called structural adjustment programs, the packages of privatization, deregulation, and trade liberalization are really designed to ensure the repayment of loans to Northern governments and commercial banks. The programs have paved the way for religious fundamentalism, human trafficking, new forms of slavery, child labor, child soldiers, child prostitutes, and the AIDS pandemic. National governments are also to blame; they are pulling out of health and education while inflating their defense budgets year after year. But this is the story of the dog chasing its own tail: structural adjustment undermines governments and opens a breach for rebels to fight guerrilla wars, which governments must buy arms to put down.

Women have organized vigorously at community, national, and international levels over the past 25 years. We participated in a succession of United Nations (UN) conferences,[1] forging an agenda of women's rights in every area of concern. We achieved success with the adoption of the Beijing Platform for Action at the Fourth World Women's Conference held in 1995, which called for women to control their own sexuality and childbearing, to be free from all forms of violence, and to have access to credit and inheritance. Since then reality has run from the rhetoric. Religious fundamentalists of every persuasion, the administration of George W. Bush foremost among them, have challenged the Beijing platform.[2] Some groups like DAWN (Development Alternatives with Women for a New Era), WGNRR (Women's Global Network for Reproductive Rights), and WEDO (Women's Environment and Development Organization) saw the danger in compromises struck with neoliberals and neo-Malthusians on the implementation plans for the Cairo Declaration and the Beijing Platform, predicting defeat and warning that the elements of neoliberal economic programs—fiscal austerity, privatization of property and services, the dismantling of welfare states, the shrinkage of government workforces and services—work against women and the fulfillment of women's health needs. Their insistent call to devote more attention to the larger structures of power that create a disabling policy environment is only now widely acted on (UNRISD 2006).

By the time of the new millennium, we were asking ourselves whether we had been pursuing the right strategies and whether the UN had the power to bring about change. The self-segregation of women in women's organizations—especially women who come from societies that are already segregated by sex—has its limitations, as the AIDS pandemic demonstrates. In parts of the global South where more women than men test positive for HIV, gender relations—meaning the power relations between men and women—are the key factor in the spread of HIV and in the impact of AIDS on women and their families. The AIDS epidemic was one of several events that challenged women to translate gender into meaningful research, analysis, and policy.

The global campaign for women's sexual and reproductive health and rights constitutes one of the strongest and most organized global feminist networks (Molyneux and Razavi 2006). This book shows why women have found it necessary to organize themselves to improve their own health. It honors the achievements of women's health movements around the world, recognizing the fight and spirit of feisty women. It is not an academic exercise. As a scholar-activist, my purpose is to record our accomplishments because they give us hope, even as they reveal what is yet to be done.

Shape of the Book

This first chapter sketches the movements for women's liberation and women's rights, women's health movements, women's fights for control of the definition of health and for understanding of the ways that subordinate gender roles complicate physical and mental medical problems. The main emphasis in this chapter, as in the book, is on women's health movements at local and national levels.[3] Women acknowledge the limitations of work at the local and national levels, where governments can usually safely ignore women's issues. Activists find the solutions to some issues lie beyond their borders, and work at the international level can give credibility to local women's activism, strengthening their voices. India, Egypt, Peru, and the United States provide the main examples of the achievements of women's activism, the obstacles that women face, the conflicts within movements, some lessons learned from the past, and some reflections on where the movements are headed. This book makes no claim to anything like a comprehensive survey of the tens of thousands of organizations around the globe that make up women's health movements. Instead it engages some of the most pressing issues that women confront and offers examples of women's groups that are organizing to find solutions.

Women's health movements exist today in a global context of inequalities between men and women and between countries of the North and South. Chapter 2 measures those inequalities and raises questions of social injustice, of the extremes of poverty that have such pernicious effects on health and longevity, and of persistent discrimination and prejudice that make poor women's lives more precarious and more miserable than those of poor men. Women's health movements strive to understand the international institutions and international agreements that dictate health conditions and determine women's access to health care. They also analyze the economic, social, and political determinants of their health, questioning standard medical authority and probing the racial and class dimensions of sexism.

Women live in multiple dimensions—in their homes, communities, and workspaces. Chapter 3 tries to answer the question, "How does the triple day—women's duties at home, in the community, and at work—affect women's health?" How does women's subordinate status limit their ability to respond to the challenges that confront them daily? Experiences of sexism filter women's activism on the job, constrain their resistance to domestic violence, and shape their responses to community issues. This chapter explores women's resistance and responses to health problems in maquilas and factories of free trade zones, the pitfalls of the work immigrants undertake far from home, the labor laws that may or may not protect them, and the specific liabilities of domestic work, sex work, and trafficking. The spread of AIDS illustrates the indivisibility of women's environments, showing how home, community, and workplace are intertwined.

All over the world women are fighting for good health services and struggling with the pharmaceutical industry. Chapter 4 describes a critical moment in women's health movements when women turn from organizing around separate issues to consider the health system as a whole and to formulate demands for health care that is responsive to all of their needs. Engaging this struggle brings women into direct confrontation with the international structures and institutions that have transformed health care in the past 25 years, commercializing both supply and expenditure. The UN Universal Declaration of Human Rights asserts that health is a human right but is silent on who has responsibility for the provision of basic health services. During the decolonization of the global South, primary responsibility fell on governments as they were the only source of sufficient resources to meet the health needs of entire populations. International development agencies are now pressing governments to turn the provision of health services over to charities, NGOs, and individual private practitioners, as part of the regressive pattern of commercialization. The specific mix of public and private care and the configuration of each nation's system remain in flux as the World Bank continues to experiment in the vast laboratory that is the global South and as the corporatization of the health sector catches up. Women's health movements are especially critical of the pharmaceutical industry and responded vigorously to breaches of ethics in medical research and clinical drug trials.

The issue of violence against women has galvanized women into action to combat domestic violence, rape, and the impunity of soldiers' wartime violence against women. Chapter 5 on the sexual politics of violence against women expands the analysis of social and interpersonal violence to considerations of economic and systemic violence and political and cultural violence against women. The emphasis is on global comparisons—honor killings as another kind of domestic violence, female genital cutting as a form of body modification, and the differences between rape in stable and war-torn societies. Women's organizations insist that all issues of violence are public, not private; that states and the international community have obligations toward women, which women have helped formulate in declarations, treaties, and conventions; that violence is a health issue as much as a social or cultural issue; and that violence against women carries very high costs.

Chapter 6 on women's reproductive health and rights follows the arguments of women's health movements around the conflicts between, on the one hand, the rights of individual women and the social groups they belong to and, on the other hand, religious dogma and national and international population control plans. Technology has transformed reproductive health care and choices, but with different consequences for women belonging to powerful groups and women in subordinated positions. Racism and class prejudice distort women's experiences; women of color everywhere are disproportionately the targets of population programs; and the state has too often manipulated technology in the interests of political objectives. Technology can be liberating; technologies for contraception and the treatment of infertility can expand women's choices and enhance their ability to control their lives. But it can also limit women's decision-making spaces and can be abused and abusive in the hands of policymakers and patriarchs. The abuse of technology leads to fetal sex selection, the commodification of body parts, and infertility treatment as a profitable business. Some women's groups are asking whether they really benefit from the new reproductive technologies, raising questions related to both gender and biology.

Movement activists are shifting the paradigm of women's health from one based on biology to one based on society. Chapter 7 reframes women's health problems by detailing two instances in which women have moved the definition of a condition out of the biomedical model and into a wider social framework: the first is disability, the second is mental illness. Although some analysts consider mental illness as a disability, others separate physical and mental conditions and compartmentalize treatment and rehabilitation for each. Yet another group insists that disablement is a universal human phenomenon, which society has systematically ignored with dire and unjust social consequences. This group argues that we need to recognize that the entire population is at risk for the concomitants of chronic illness and disability, that disability is an infinitely various but universal feature of the human condition. We need a political strategy that demystifies the specialness of disability, and the principles of universal design must apply everywhere; otherwise we risk pitting the disabled with their special needs, wants, and rights against the rest of the population in a world of finite resources. The disability rights movement has spread from the North to the South where war, poverty, and poor care in pregnancy and childbirth create ever-larger populations of disabled children and adults. Stereotypes exaggerate the condition of disabled women and by sexism and bias, constrain their life chances beyond the limits of their handicap. The dearth of resources in the South calls for a new universalist approach, one that leapfrogs the slow evolution of a more comprehensive policy in the North. The philosophical core lies in a new tolerance of diversity and a resistance to a conformity that dictates a single standard of beauty. South and North, women must challenge neoliberalism, eugenics, racism, and new forms of discrimination against immigrants, women, the disabled, and the aged.

Movements for Women's Liberation
and Women's Rights

Women's movements have many antecedents in other struggles and many foremothers, those outspoken women who challenged what seemed immutable, often at great personal cost. For every country with a women's movement, the list of predecessors includes general mobilizations like struggles for abolition, suffrage, and trade unions as well as against colonial rule, and specific fights for women's rights and women's health. This section opens with a brief discussion of social movements and advocacy to situate women's movements in the universe of social movements and to distinguish social movements from NGOs. An outline of several national women's movements follows, to give a sense of how women organized and how they addressed the issues of their day: examples are drawn from India, Egypt, Peru, and the United States.

Social Movements for Progressive Social Change

Social movements comprise networks of informal interactions that tie together informal groups and individuals, and sometimes formal organizations, in struggles for social change on the basis of a shared identity (Eschle and Stammers 2000).[4] Peggy Antrobus (2004), a leading Caribbean feminist, believes women's movements do not conform to this profile because they lack common objectives, continuity, and unity, and because they are crosscutting; some focus on gender identity, others on social transformation—all are political and reject patriarchal privilege. Sociologists generally base theories of social movements on European and North American evidence, casting the middle class as leaders of the new social movements and finding participants concerned with the values of autonomy and identity (Pichardo 1997). In contrast Latin American commentators observe that people at the lowest rung of the socioeconomic ladder—the excluded and the marginalized—are the central protagonists of current struggles for social justice (Zibechi 2005). Sociological theory generally accounts for "left-wing" movements but not counter or conservative movements (for example, militia, right-to-life, and Christian right movements) (Pichardo 1997). This omission sets up a left-right binary of social movements from which nongovernmental organizations may be exempt and thereby depoliticized.

Women's movements are, roughly, of three types: human rights ("nonpolitical" protest movements), popular women's movements (formed for mutual support), and feminist movements (led by middle-class and professional women) (UNRISD 2000).[5] Whether reform movements (focused on legal change) or radical movements (focused on changing values and norms), women's movements advocate for improvements in women's status; they monitor the impact of public and private sector activities on women; and they provide services for women. Body politics—which clusters struggles around gender violence, sexual choice, reproductive rights, and women's health—is the focus that distinguishes women's rights movements from other rights movements (Harcourt 2006). Organizations represent the active component of social movements but are not the movements themselves, although the distinction between women's organizations and women's movements is not clearcut. A majority of professional activists view themselves as part of women's movements, and the organizations that activists belong to vary in their power, resources, ideology, and relations to donors and governments, as well as in the extent and quality of their connections with grassroots movements.

Many organizations that identify themselves as part of the women's movement have common characteristics: national in scope, controlled by women, feminist in outlook, led by consumers, and engaged in advocacy, service, and education. Despite these commonalities the structure of these organizations varies greatly: some are large, centralized, and hierarchical; some are small, decentralized, and participatory; and some combine characteristics of both types. Some groups are nationwide and linked to international networks (for example, organizationally as chapters); some are community based and local. Some employ staff and are financially dependent on government or external support; some are self-financed and run entirely by volunteers. Some start informally as groups of like-minded individuals; some are the idea of a single person.

When movement members work within the system as researchers, policy planners, and advocates, divided loyalties may result. Advocacy needs explanation and definition. What makes an advocate, according to Sofia Montenegro, one of the prime movers of the (Nicaraguan) National Women's Coalition,[6] is the ability to synthesize and organize academic knowledge and political experience and give it back so that others can use it in their fights; advocates are those women in a third world country who have the privilege to access information and are willing to use it in this way (Connell 2001). HERA, which stands for Health, Empowerment, Rights and Accountability, is an international network of women's health advocates; it defines advocacy as, "a strategic, long-term process founded on analysis and goal-setting to bring about change within a system" (Abdullah 2003, 35). For the Centre for Development and Population Activities (CEDPA) based in Washington, DC, a nonprofit international organization founded in 1975 to provide access to high quality reproductive health and voluntary family planning, advocacy is speaking up, drawing attention to an important issue, and directing decision makers toward a solution.

Activities that would build and strengthen women's movements face acute problems in obtaining funds. A study by AWID (2005), the Association for Women's Rights in Development, found that 51 percent of women's organizations are receiving less funding than they were in 2000. In the Asian region, women's groups lack funds for exchange programs among plantation and migrant women, documentation, development of new leadership, and meetings to strategize around globalization, militarization, and migration. In an acute commentary on global feminist advocacy, Charkiewicz (2004) observes that from the early 1990s social movements, including feminist movements, metamorphosed into NGOs, an organizational form that draws on the corporate model; the effect is to delink social movements from the grassroots, which effectively depoliticizes women. The "NGO-ization" of feminism in Latin America gradually professionalized the work of activists, creating networks, concentrating resources, and accentuating their specialized character in various ways, including by sectors (Barrig 1999).

Donors propelled some of the change from movement to NGO. In Chile many women's NGOs closed projects that were closely associated with their feminist commitments—such as popular education projects on sexuality and parenting, and leadership training—and in order to remain economically viable they opened projects that are more attractive to funders, like activities dealing with women's health, micro-enterprise development, and job training for women heads of household (UNRSID 2000). NGOs that use charity from the wealthy as a solution to major social problems such as unemployment that working class women face represent a return to what Hatem (1995, 236) calls "the old piecemeal patronization of the poor."

Feminists did not invent the format of NGOs engaging the UN system as stakeholders representing the interests of different groups (Charkiewicz 2004). The UN determines the interests in frameworks that are not up for negotiation. As a result UN documents may adopt language proposed by women, but the UN system leaves power regimes intact. Women gain a voice but not power or influence. The UN's failure to implement the promises of various action plans explains why so many women's groups feel they have been losing ground since the Fourth World Women's Conference held in Beijing in 1995.

A review of NGOs in the Middle East confirms Charkiewicz's observation that institutions and movements have reincarnated as NGOs. In the 1990s, three trends converged to drive the exponential growth of NGOs in the Middle East: economic trends such as the international financial institutions' shift from government loans to nongovernmental grants; social trends like the elevation of human rights, environmental justice, and feminism to cosmopolitan concerns; and such political trends as governments' suppression of oppositional political parties and greater license to religious and charitable organizations (Carapico 2000). In Palestine NGOs had their origins in mass mobilizations and the national front strategy; grassroots organizing comprised nonfactional groups of women, students, and workers. Those seeking an alternative to the Palestine National Authority initially embraced NGOs but later came to see them as an employment sector of the economically privileged (Hammami 2000).

The change from social movements to nongovernmental organizations has occurred in the context of globalization (discussed in chapter 2) and a political climate of increased poverty, growing religious fundamentalism, and entrenched militarism. Grassroots work becomes more difficult in this altered climate, and the professional NGOs coopt the space for a movement-building approach to social change. The current state of women's movements reflects all of these changes.

Those who favor NGOs identify them with civil society and associate the support of NGOs with the promotion of civil society and an agenda for good governance. Libertarians, who value freedom above equality, represent NGOs as civil society's attempt to liberate citizens from the grip of the state. Donors—international organizations, bilateral aid programs, and large foundations—believe NGOs represent popular struggles for democracy. They portray NGOs as the key to development from below, and they borrow leading words like "indigenous" and "grassroots" from radical and populist critiques of the state to contrast this path with (implicitly bad) state-led "elitist" development practices of the past. In this portrait donors are conflating bigness and bureaucracy, turning the "small-is-beautiful" argument into an attack on the state. Neoliberals limit the definition of civil society by excluding trade unions and then representing NGOs as a foil for international institutions seeking to discredit the state by attacking state power and manipulating civil society. The assault on the state contradicts the rhetoric of democracy, transparency, and efficiency, because the private sector is certainly none of those things (Amin 1995). (For a full discussion of the contributions and failures of NGOs to health services see Turshen 1999.)

Women's organizations founded in the 1990s are professionalized and rarely integral to broader movements for social change. Not surprisingly, as their leaders tend to be highly trained physicians and scientists, women's health organizations tend to be about a single disease. Their concern is to make their educated constituencies aware of medical and scientific information, and they focus on ensuring women an equitable share of psychological, social, and biological science and treatment (Ruzek and Becker 1999). They also accept corporate sponsorship, which an earlier generation of movement organizers would have found compromising.

El-Gawhary (2000, 39), writing about Egypt, also found that the new NGOs are professionalized, staffed by well educated and highly trained activists ("social and political élites"); their priorities are women's issues, democratization, and human rights, but they are divorced from the realities of the rural poor and they lack popular support. She calls these the "advocacy NGOs" and says that generous foreign funding helps them in their mission to challenge the Mubarak government. The local press sometimes covers their activities, but their main audience seems to be foreign embassies and the international conference circuit; "this has not yet translated into desired change."

From 2000, as faith in the UN agenda as a meaningful medium for social change collapsed in the conferences that reviewed progress since Rio, Vienna, Cairo, and Beijing, women's movements began to engage with broader economic justice movements that were addressing unfair trade, odious debt, the dark side of globalization, and the imperious role of the international financial institutions (Harcourt 2006). Regional organizing and meeting in social forums outside UN venues took on new significance. Protests galvanized around organizations like the G-8 and the World Trade Organization, which were not part of the UN system.

National Women's Movements

The global history of national women's movements belies the accusation frequently brought by opponents that feminism is a Western concept, alien to their societies and cultures. Many women's movements date back to the eighteenth and nineteenth centuries: four stand out—the Indian women's movement, still among the most vibrant and influential in the world; the Egyptian women's movement, which is struggling to maintain its early accomplishments; the Peruvian women's movement, which has steadily confronted a hostile environment; and the U.S. women's movement, which has lost so much ground in recent years. Race, class, caste, and religious issues dominated the early feminist movements in Egypt, India, Peru, and the United States and conditioned their engagement in abolitionist, anticolonial, and nationalist movements as well as in struggles to improve women's status. Participation was often personally costly, and nonwhite, lower class, and lower caste women paid more heavily than elite women.

India

Indian women were involved in politics from the late eighteenth century when impoverished women and men staged famine revolts against British colonialists (Swarup et al. 1994). In the nineteenth century high caste women campaigned for women's education and against harmful practices like female infanticide, child marriage, widow immolation, and the ban on widow remarriage. In the early twentieth century women like Saroj Nalini Dutt (1887–1924) and Saraladevi Chaudhurani (1872–1945) founded women's committees and women's institutes, some local and some national in scope. From 1904 to 1911 women activists took part in the Swadeshi movement for self-sufficiency, which called for the boycott of British goods and the substitution of home-spun *khadi* cloth, and from 1918 to 1922 in Non-Cooperation, a movement of protests, strikes, and other acts of civil resistance led by Mohandas Gandhi (1869–1948) (Everett 1979).

An early success of the Women's India Association was limited suffrage for women in the 1919 Government of India Act (Swarup et al. 1994). Sarojini Naidu (1879–1949) became the first woman president of the Indian National Congress in 1925 and she was the first woman to join Gandhi's 1930 Salt March to circumvent the British monopoly on mining and taxing salt by producing and selling sea salt (Butalia 1997). From 1930 to 1934 women were prominent among the hundreds of thousands that picketed British establishments (Gandhi's Civil Disobedience movement), and from 1942 until independence in 1947 women campaigned for the Quit India movement, with many serving time in jail. Upper class and upper caste women had preferred legislative debates to nonviolent mass movements until Sarojini Naidu linked freedom for women with freedom for India and brought the two movements together. Differences persisted on the issue of women's role in society, an ideological conflict "between those who looked to the pristine purity of an idealized past, when women and men had separate but complementary roles, and those who saw the reality of women's multidimensional roles" (Swarup et al. 1994, 367).

Independence brought constitutional guarantees of justice, liberty, equality, and individual dignity, freeing women to shift their attention to reform of personal laws that governed marriage, divorce, and property rights. After the fierce fight for the Hindu Code Bills,[7] women's groups turned to the implementation of social welfare measures. The movements of the 1970s shed light on women's new campaigns and preoccupations (violence, food, work, and governance). The Shahada was a movement of Bhil tribal landless laborers against the exploitive practices of nontribal local landowners; rising militancy among women turned it into a campaign against alcohol-fueled domestic violence, leading women "to storm liquor dens and destroy liquor pots" (Kumar 1995, 61). The Self-Employed Women's Association in Gujarat was the first attempt to form a women's trade union among poorly paid women working in bad conditions, harassed by authorities and the police. Also in Gujarat, women agitated against rising prices, forming the United Women's Anti Price Rise Front, which they turned into a consumer protection campaign that even housebound women participated in (by coordinated demonstrations of thousands of women banging rolling pins on metal plates). The Front evolved into the New Light (*Nav Nirman*), a massive middle-class movement joined by thousands of women to protest prices, black marketeering, and corruption, which in turn became an all-out criticism of the Indian State (Kumar 1995). By 1974 the women of Hyderabad had formed the Progressive Organization of Women, "the first women's group associated with the contemporary feminist movement," followed the next year by "the sudden development of a whole spate of feminist activities in Maharashtra" (Kumar 1995, 62–63).

An autobiographical note by T.K. Sundari Ravindran (1997, 18), a participant in these events, vividly illustrates the motives of young Indian women.

The early 1970s, my university years, were a period of turmoil in India. Peasant uprisings, the armed struggle of urban youth against the state, general strikes in essential sectors, declaration of political emergency by a ruling party unable to contain public discontent, and mass mobilization against this onslaught on democracy—these and more marked this period. By the time I had completed six years of university, I had moved on from being a do-good community volunteer to an adult educator engaged in "conscientisation" of the rural poor from the dalit communities, the lowest in the caste hierarchy.

I was 24 and an activist from a small rural women's group in South India when I attended the 3rd International Women and Health Meeting (IWHM) in Geneva in June 1981. . . . The meeting inspired new ideas and exposed me to the feminist critique of the medicalisation of women's health. One of the most important outcomes of the third IWHM for me and our group was the challenge to evolve our own analysis of the structural causes underlying the ill health of poor women in developing countries. . . . The rural women's group, which I co-founded with 12 local dalit women, is going strong 16 years on. . . . The struggle for women's reproductive rights was and continues to be for the group an essential component of the larger struggle for social justice.

Egypt

The Egyptian women's movement began in the nineteenth century with upper class women in urban areas; Huda Sha'rawi (1879–1947) and Duriya Shafiq (1908–1975) are among the best known early feminists, but many other women expressed a feminist consciousness in their writings. Some also engaged with liberal men in a debate about "the woman question,"[8] considering such issues as seclusion, segregation, and veiling (Guenena and Wassef 1999). In the early part of the twentieth century, women like Malak Hifni Nassef (1886–1918) began to demand that the Egyptian Nationalist Congress grant women access to education and professional opportunities and that they reform the personal status laws that regulated marriage, divorce, and child custody (Guenena and Wassef 1999). Health concerns were immediately on the agenda: maternal and child health services, tuberculosis treatment, provision of clean water, and prevention of water-borne diseases like schistosomiasis (a parasite carried by snails) and cholera (Badran 1995). Efforts to eradicate female circumcision, a nearly universal practice in Egypt, date from the 1920s (Al-Dawla 2000). Women participated in the 1919 Revolution, a movement for Egypt's independence from Great Britain,[9] and even joined in street demonstrations that turned into riots. Police response differentiated upper class women whom they sexually harassed from lower class women several of whom they killed (Guenena and Wassef 1999). In 1923 Huda Sha'rawi and ten other women founded the Egyptian Feminist Union, issuing 32 demands that included nationalist, social, educational, and economic reforms as well as women's equality (Badran 1995). By the 1930s the women's movement had spread and the number of organizations multiplied, though they split along class lines (middle class women split from upper class women) and in the 1960s middle class women split along religious lines (Islamists against secular groups). The new demands were equality before the law and political representation (The New Woman Research and Study Center 1996).

From 1954, with the departure of the British, the ascension of Gamal Abdel Nasser, and the creation of a socialist state, Egyptian women gained equal rights in employment and education; in 1956 they gained the right to vote and run for elected office, and in the 1970s reform of personal status laws. Hatem (1994) stresses the unique role of the state in women's lives in this period and the phenomenon of state feminism, which from the 1960s transformed working class and middle class women into dependent clients of the state. For example, dependence on the state undermined the viability of women candidates for political office, and without an independent political base, women had no power to determine state policies regarding their representation. The creation of women's NGOs as an alternative to state feminism began in the late 1970s. Two organizations, the Mansura-based Daughter of the Land Association and the Cairo-based Solidarity of Arab Women's Association, addressed the growing Islamist-led conservatism of Egyptian society.

One of the best-known feminists to have written about sexuality in Egypt is Nawal El Saadawi (1999, 291–292). In her autobiography, she describes her activism:

> As a rural doctor I lived close to village people, shared their experiences, learnt about their lives, witnessed what the triple scourge of poverty, ignorance and sickness did to them. Women bore a double burden since they also suffered from the oppression exercised on them by father and husbands, brothers and uncles and other men. I saw young girls burn themselves alive, or throw themselves into the waters of the Nile and drown, in order to escape a father's, or a husband's tyranny. I tried to help them but the men with power in the village in agreement with the state authorities had me transferred somewhere else, accusing me of not

respecting the traditional values of their community, of inciting women to rebel against religion and its laws.

I was not attracted by the medical profession. It seemed unable to do much in the face of the sufferings imposed on people. I realized how sickness and poverty are linked to politics, to money and power, that medical practice was removed from our everyday life. Writing became a weapon with which to fight the system, which draws its authority from the autocratic power exercised by the ruler of the state, and that of the father or the husband in the family. The written word for me became an act of rebellion against injustice exercised in the name of religion, or morals, or love.

Peru

Peruvian women first organized politically in the 1920s to demand the vote; their bid was unsuccessful as the 1933 constitution did not give the vote to women or to peasants. The gulf between the law and reality enabled the oligarchical state to deny women's capacity as individuals and their right to citizenship. Women won the right to vote in 1955, more as a result of military leaders courting women's endorsement than of pressure from women. Modernization and urbanization in the 1950s strengthened civil society in a country fragmented by cultural, ethnic, linguistic, and regional differences and polarized by extremes of wealth and poverty (Vargas and Villanueva 1994).

The Velasco regime (1968–1975) established in Peru in 1968 reacted against the ruling class and not against popular classes. The regime installed a set of social and economic reforms based on leftist ideology through strengthening the Communist Party and developing close relations with unions, shantytowns, and the universities. However, the methods of social control based on repression, persecution, and restriction of civil and political freedoms were similar to those used in undemocratic countries like Chile, Argentina, Uruguay, and Brazil. New social actors emerged in Peru: women, young people, and a revitalized Catholic Church. When the military government instituted economic austerity in the late 1970s and early 1980s, an alliance of women, youth, and Liberation theologians turned against the dictatorship. These groups did not call for a return to democratic political institutions, as they did not interpret them as beneficial for the masses, but instead demanded better salaries and the satisfaction of basic needs (Padilla 2004).

Since 1973, when the collective *Acción para la Liberación de la Mujer Peruana* (ALIMUPER, Action for the Liberation of Peruvian Women) organized a march protesting the use of the female body in beauty contests (which was reported in a local newspaper under the title "The Rebellion of the Witches"), the nascent Peruvian feminist movement has campaigned against the commercialization of the body and maternity, linking the two to women's reproductive rights. In 1979, an ALIMU-PER manifesto called for a feminist demonstration with three major goals: the legalization of abortion, access to birth control, and opposition to forced sterilization. "These three issues," says the manifesto, "can only be dealt with together: all have to do with alienation of our bodies" (Barrig 1999, 6).

In 1978 the Movement Manuela Ramos, a nonprofit feminist organization, opened an office in Lima dedicated to advocacy, investigation, and the defense of economic and social rights; eventually it reached over 600,000 women belonging to the diverse cultures living in Peru. The movement organized projects along four thematic themes: economic rights to a life without violence; women's human rights; political rights; and sexual and reproductive citizenship and rights. Growing from a small grassroots organization to a regional leader in battling violence against women and increasing women's economic independence and political participation, the *Movimiento Manuela Ramos* carried out pioneering work with rural indigenous women in the Peruvian Amazon. This work became a regional model for grassroots participatory research; it enabled women to identify their own reproductive health needs and priorities, which guided the development of community health projects.

Fernando Belaunde regained power (1980–1985) and reinstalled democratic government. The economic crisis was so severe that food and other goods started arriving from different international development agencies. At the same time that women and neighborhood associations started organizing, the government began the distribution of food, enforcing an *asistencialista* welfare state model, which had implications for women's strategy and actions. New types of organizations gained visibility throughout the country: communal kitchen, the glass of milk, mothers' clubs, medical stands, and child-care centers for working mothers.

In 1985, Alan Garcia from the APRA party (American Popular Revolutionary Alliance) became president, implementing a populist government and continuing the previous welfare state model with new populist characteristics. "The APRA government (1985–1990) saw women's organizations—such as the 2000 mothers' clubs created under a program headed by Alan Garcia's wife—as a promising arena for co-optation and clientelistic politics" (Barrig 1994, 171). In 1990,

Alberto Fujimori was elected to office and in 1992, he pulled off a self-coup d'état or *autogolpe* that closed down the Peruvian Congress and launched a package of economic reforms based on neoliberal policies. The new policies strongly affected the working class, women, and the poor. Women's organizations of the 1990s are a product of those political and economic developments (Barrig 1994; Padilla 2004).[10]

Peruvian women from many walks of life joined the women's movement in the 1970s; here is one account by Magda Mateus Cardenas, Director of Centro Amauta, Cusco, Peru (quoted in Sweetman 1997, 62):

> My life has been influenced by circumstances, other people, and a multitude of challenges. I believe that in this I am similar to many women who have come from a less privileged background than mine. In the 1970s, I was one of many young people of my generation who wanted change, and became politically active. I learned to read Marxist texts, and take a look at the reality of my country. I didn't have to go without food or housing, but I remember learning that there were many social and economic disparities in this country, that marked you out; they made one want to do something with one's life, in order to escape them. In the 1980s I was the first woman to become president of the Centro Federado de Estudiantes de Antropolgía (Federation of Anthropology Students) . . . Eventually I joined Centro Amauta, a feminist organisation, with which I still work today. The experience of the Amauta team was something new for me; it touched on many points I was not aware of previously, including sexual and reproductive rights, and the problem of violence against women. Over the years that I have worked with the team, we have expanded our perspectives and our commitments, until we are now an organisation which is consulted on issues of gender, class, and culture at both national and regional level.

The United States

The U.S. experience presented here exemplifies the ongoing nature of struggles for women's health; indeed many of us feel we are fighting the same battles over and over again, even as we win legal, political, and social changes.

American and British women took active roles on both sides of the eighteenth-century revolutionary war as soldiers, spies, nurses, cooks, and laundresses. They also joined abolitionist movements, in America from 1775 and in Great Britain from 1787.[11] The first wave of the U.S. women's movement emerged in the 1840s about the same time as the Popular Health Movement, which was a social movement to redefine disease as preventable by people (as opposed to a divinity or an elitist physician); women's heath was one component of the Popular Health Movement. By the 1870s the women's movement turned on the issues of voluntary motherhood, sex education, and birth control. These early feminists were suffragists and moral reformers, and some were advocates of free love (Gordon 1977). The modern birth control movement, with its beliefs in reproductive self-determination and sexual indulgence, emerged in the early twentieth century with a call for a transformation of women's rights. The second wave of the U.S. women's movement in the 1960s made many of the same demands and had a similar vision: the leading health issues were the imperative need for legalized contraception and abortion and an end to sterilization abuse.

The new women's liberation movement built on other movements of the 1960s like the peace movement, the antinuclear movements (against the atomic bomb and against nuclear energy plants), the anti-Vietnam war movement (which put women in touch with anti-imperialist groups in the Third World), science for the people and popular epidemiology, the 1965 Berkeley free speech movement, and at the end of the decade, the gay liberation movement. From these movements women learned to question authority, especially medical authority, and to put personal issues into a social and political context. Women relearned the techniques of nonviolent mass mobilization based on the need to organize public and collective protests. They also learned the value of politics, policymaking, and the important role of the state in their lives, lessons already known to women in Europe, Africa, Asia, and Latin America, where government services supported so many women.

The new U.S. women's movement was made up of two distinct strands—radical feminists who came out of the New Left and the Civil Rights movement and mainstream, middle-class, mainly white women, led by Betty Freidan, the founder of NOW (the National Organization of Women). Judy MacLean (1980, 242) writes,

We needed both, and the women's movement became a mass movement only because we had both. We needed the daring, the vision, the radical questioning of every aspect of our lives. But we also needed the concern for institutions, for legislation and court cases that the reformers provided. NOW was able to capture much of the radical energy that was too explosive for the women's liberation groups precisely because NOW had the formal structure and large membership the others considered unfeminist. But it would have been lacking in élan and direction without the new left women's groups.

The Civil Rights Act of 1964 prohibited discrimination or segregation in regards to voting and employment; in the case of the latter the Act specifically extended its protections to women (http://usinfo.state.gov/ usa/infousa/laws/majorlaw/civilr19.htm accessed 10 June 2006). In 1966 NOW persuaded the Equal Employment Opportunity Commission, newly established to combat job discrimination, to take the sex discrimination clause seriously. NOW won the executive order that has been the basis for affirmative action for women who work for companies that do business with the federal government. The organization put an end to help-wanted ads that separated men and women; and they defended airline attendants (then known as "stewardesses") who wanted to work past age 30.

For many of us, the history of the women's health movement is embodied in the experience of the Boston Women's Health Book Collective.

The history of Our Bodies, Ourselves and the Boston Women's Health Book Collective (BWHBC) began in the spring of 1969 at a women's liberation conference held in Boston. At a workshop on "Women and their Bodies," we discovered that every one of us had a "doctor story," that we had all experienced feelings of frustration and anger toward to medical maze in general, and toward those doctors who were condescending, paternalistic, judgmental and uninformative in particular. As we talked and shared our experiences, we realized just how much we had to learn about our bodies, that simply finding a "good doctor" was not the solution to whatever problems we might have. So we decided on a summer project: we would research our questions, share what we learned in our group, and then present the information in the fall as a course "by and for women." We envisioned an ongoing process that would involve other women who would then go on to teach such a course in other settings. . . .

The founders of BWHBC were all college educated, but a significant number of us were from working-class backgrounds and were the first in our families to attend college. Some of us had professional degrees, but none of us were in health fields. Many of us had been active in the social protest movements of the 1960s, particularly the civil rights movement, the antiwar movement, movements for women-centered childbirth and legal abortion. Some of us came from families with histories of struggle for social justice. Others of us came of age during a time of social change and found our own way to political activism. When we came together as part of a larger women's liberation movement, we were thrilled by the realization that working for social justice could affect the conditions of our lives as women. We believed that with our newfound freedom and solidarity as feminists, we could be more effective advocates on behalf of ourselves and other women, as well as other progressive causes. (Judy Diskin Norsigian et al. 2000)

Obstacles Women Confront and their Resistance

Women's movements face obstacles and resistance to their demands is in evidence everywhere; in some cases the opposition amounts to a backlash against previous gains. In the 1970s and 1980s, neoliberal economic ideology committed the International Monetary Fund and the World Bank to stabilization and structural adjustment as the basis for economic recovery from recession and for long-term economic growth; this philosophy, which has instigated a damaging assault on women's welfare, continues to dominate international development policy and practice. At the same time as international financial organizations were imposing their "reforms," the women's movement appeared on the international stage in the International Decade for Women (1976–1985). One interpretation of this coincidental timing is that increasing hardships caused by the rising cost of living forced women to confront economic realities (Daines and Seddon 1993), and the UN provided a convenient forum to share experiences. Another reading of the events suggests that the UN assisted women's movements by providing them with an international platform because women's nongovernmental organizations served as an escape valve in a period of extensive resistance and widespread rioting. "Bread riots," also known as "IMF riots," were the most dramatic form of collective popular protest against austerity; women took part in such riots in Dominican Republic, Egypt, Indonesia, Jamaica, Jordan, Peru, Tunisia, Venezuela, and elsewhere.

One of the earliest groups of women from the global South, DAWN responded to structural adjustment programs by promoting a feminist perspective on development. An international South-South network, DAWN addressed economic structures and the environment as priority concerns, along with women's reproductive rights. Other international networks like Women Living under Muslim Laws, founded in 1984, included reproductive rights as a significant component of its research (Garcia-Moreno and Claro 1994).

Working in the international arena brought rewards and resources to national women's movements but they paid a high price: conformity to the international agenda and the sacrifice of local issues much closer to the interests of women at the base, especially in rural areas. In the early years of the International Decade for Women, Northern groups assumed women's interests were everywhere the same, as they shared common conditions of oppression. Attitudes changed as Southern women stepped forward and asserted their diverse positions. International relations between social movements, advocacy groups, and NGOs are still not always smooth or productive. A politically effective women's movement experiences pressure from single-issue, foreign-funded NGOs; proliferating NGOs exert pressure in a direction opposite to that of local and national women's movements, toward the compartmentalization of particular needs and problems and away from a movement-building approach to social change. "Our main task is to develop a discourse that is an alternative to the fundamentalists," said Rita Giacaman, Director of the Department of International Community Health at Bir Zeit University and a Palestinian community health activist; "with all due respect to Western feminists—their work is very helpful but it suffers from serious problems as far as we're concerned, for example, the lack of the notion of nationhood as instrumental to any analysis. Here, this is crucial. We need to develop our own theoretical conceptions of what gender is in the Palestinian context." (quoted in Connell 2001, 152)

Relations with national governments pose as many problems as working in the international arena. In India, the state has used the women's movement and drawn upon the strengths of its activists to gain access to women living invisibly in feudal households. Women's movement activists challenged basic feudal and patriarchal structures and succeeded in bringing women out of oppressive family structures. The state recognized this as a necessary prerequisite for the acceptance of population control measures. Activists in the women's movements wondered whether they had really changed women's lives, even as they knew they had widened women's roles (Sawhney 1999).

In South Africa, problems with the government arose at the end of the apartheid era when women expected fruitful cooperation. Rural South African women had long experience in self-organization prior to and separate from the liberation struggle, through such community institutions as burial societies and savings clubs, and they built on this experience during the antiapartheid struggle. Organizations like the Natal Organization of Women, based in Durban, the Federation of Transvaal Women around Johannesburg, and the United Women's Organization in the Western Cape ran workshops on domestic and communal violence and developed rape crisis networks, among other activities. But after 1990, when the South African government unbanned the African National Congress (ANC), these organizations voluntarily merged with the ANC-sponsored Women's League, which dropped many of the women's innovative self-help programs. The merger demobilized grassroots women, and in response women created the Women's National Coalition in 1992 to draft a charter of women's rights that would inform the legal structures of the new South Africa. Once that work was completed, the Women's League tried to block attempts at further independent organizing (Connell 2001).

The Filipino Women's Movement has assessed its difficulties: relations with the state are tenuous, somewhere between tentative collaboration and outright opposition. Filipinas say that two decades of organizing have yielded three clear gains. First, gender is now visible and legitimate, no longer dismissed in policy discussions, which now include rape, domestic violence, and reproductive rights. Second, gender advocacy has moved from the capital to the provinces and from the academies to sites of daily life in workplaces, urban slums, and rural farms. Third, women have learned to build healing facilities—women's clinics, women's crisis centers, community programs to combat domestic violence, and women's micro-enterprises (Pilipina 1995).

In addition to obstacles coming from outside the women's movements, difficulties arise around issues of reform, class, ethics, and finances. Pilipina, a mass-based feminist organization working for women's full participation in leadership and governance in the Philippines, openly acknowledges internal dilemmas around working with traditional women's organizations. Traditionalists in the Philippines women's movement are silent on the need to challenge the economic, social, and political status quo. In contrast, Pilipina says that their struggle runs along class as well as gender lines, and that they do not aspire merely to put more women into positions of power without any prospect of real and lasting structural change (Pilipina 1995).

Freeing themselves from the tutelage of political parties without becoming isolated is a major challenge for feminists in countries like Eritrea emerging from liberation struggles. And for women in Morocco and Turkey, successful autonomy depends on extending their social base to a more diverse constituency, but as yet there are too few signs of such cross-class alliances (UNRISD 2000). Other internal dilemmas of women's groups turn on ethical questions such as integrity, transparency, and honesty in claiming credit for work done; competition for funds; and the careerism of a few feminists and women advocates who make careers out of consultancies at the expense of movement work that brings minimal financial rewards.

The National Union of Eritrean Women (NUEW), originally founded under the auspices of the Eritrean People's Liberation Front, successfully reconstituted as an autonomous social movement in 1992. NUEW spearheaded changes in the civil code inherited from Ethiopia: now marriage contracts can be made only with the full consent of both parties; the law raises the age of eligibility for marriage from 15 to 18 years; it recognizes both mothers and fathers as family heads; it bans discrimination between men and women in divorce cases; it extends paid maternity leave from 45 to 60 days; it legalizes abortion in cases of threat to maternal mental or physical health, rape or incest; and it extends the mandatory sentence for rape to 15 years (Connell 2001). In 1994, some members of NUEW called for formal bans on premarital virginity testing, female circumcision, and infibulation (a more severe form of genital cutting); they asked that domestic violence become grounds for divorce and that the civil code cover all Eritreans, including Muslim women ruled by *shari'a* law (Connell 2001, 119).

Women are involved in everyday forms of resistance to government and powerful figures that run their lives; everyday forms of resistance are as important as the more overt and organized forms of cooperative and collective struggle (Daines and Seddon 1993). Everyday defiance includes passive resistance, individual self-help (survival strategies), and struggles over unequal control and distribution of resources between women and men in households. Women may refuse to cooperate with health services—to attend, to follow advice, to obtain prescribed drugs—behavior that health workers mistakenly ascribe to women's ignorance, failing to see the rebellion in these acts.

Women's Health Movements

Body politics are at the heart of what distinguishes women's rights movements from other rights movements—the struggles to end gender violence, ensure sexual choice, and promote reproductive rights and women's health (Harcourt 2006).

The forerunners of today's women's health movements are the European public health movements of the eighteenth and nineteenth centuries: the early work of the French revolution, Bismarckians of the 1848 revolution in Germany, and that of reformers reacting to the health crises created by the Industrial Revolution and sudden urbanization. The history of health care over the twentieth century is that of recurrent political struggle: commercial health care has expanded; political struggles have constrained it; and corporations and international organizations are promoting it anew in countries at all levels of development (Mackintosh 2003). Public health workers are by definition in favor of government services. Public health has always been a reform movement, attracting progressive people to confront the medical profession and leaders of the business community, to prod governments into protecting the poor, mothers and children, workers, the disabled, the aged, and disadvantaged people of color.

Reformers in the English sanitary movement protested against the short, miserable lives of the urban poor and brought about the first public health acts, the first labor laws protecting child workers, the first laws requiring inspection of workplaces, the first building and housing codes, and more. Just as nineteenth-century reformers opposed liberal laissez-faire economic philosophies, twentieth-century reformers opposed neoliberal versions of those philosophies (the Washington Consensus, embodied in the international financial institutions that dictate privatization, cutbacks in government social programs, deregulation, and cutting taxes).

The "public" in public health refers first to government services, usually paid for out of general tax revenues rather than by the users of services at the facility. Second, governments provide services in public spaces to which everyone has access in principle. Third, public means the community, not the individual: public health protects the community from hazards to which everyone is exposed. For example, large numbers of people benefit from iodized salt to prevent goiter (McNeil 2006). Public health measures are usually preventive and collective; in contrast, clinical medical care is usually curative and individual.

Public space is also political space, and it is impossible to underestimate the importance of political climate to women's health movements. Social movements depend on government guarantees of freedom of speech and assembly; paradoxically, social movements often oppose those very governments. During the 1980s, a period of political liberalism in Brazil, women's groups pushed for and won the creation of state councils for women's rights, giving feminists a solid base from which to develop and propose government health initiatives (Soares et al. 1995). The federal government created the Integrated Program for Women's Health and incorporated the right to family planning in the Brazilian constitution. After the change of government in 1989, implementation of these programs became sporadic.

Women's health movements position themselves in relation to science and medicine, arguing with scientists about issues of scientific truth and scientific method and with physicians about the efficacy and style of their care. Women seek to reform science and medicine by exerting pressure from the outside, by training as scientists and doctors in ever-greater numbers to exert pressure from within, and by locating themselves in academic, research, and policy establishments. Women health activists question the uses, control, and contents of science and medicine as well as the processes by which scientists produce the contents. Movement activists claim to speak credibly as experts in their own right, as people who know about scientific matters and who can contribute to the discourse on truth.[12] By establishing themselves as experts women try to change the ground rules on how researchers conduct their scientific work and how doctors practice medicine. Ultimately, women's health movements seek to democratize science, demanding that scientific elites and institutions respond to community concerns, that the public participate in setting research priorities, that the medical–industrial complex submit to popular control, and that medical science reorganize to facilitate universal access to health care (Epstein 1991). Women's groups also fight the medicalization of social problems, which is a trap entailed in the transfer of technology from North to South. Some bureaucrats in government health ministries acquiesce in using medical interventions to try to solve problems that they could better avoid through social changes. Educated women's health activists are also conscious of their roles as translators, of the need to demystify highly technical medical information, and convey it in languages accessible to most women.

Starting a women's health movement is difficult: even in the United States, where literacy is almost universal, public libraries are well stocked, and tools like the Freedom of Information Act enable researchers to penetrate realms of secrecy, women find it very hard to access key materials. These investigative tasks are far more difficult in other countries. It is nearly impossible, for example, to get unbiased information on treatments and pharmaceuticals in places where the lack of constraints on transnational corporations makes them virtually unaccountable to any government agency, let alone the public (Yanco 1996).

Despite the difficulties, women's health movements have grown dramatically since the 1980s, and today the movements are large and dynamic. International organizations like Isis International, created in 1974 as an information and communication channel for women, is part of a global network of about 50,000 contacts in 150 countries. The Women's Global Network for Reproductive Rights (WGNRR), the International Women's Health Coalition, and groups like the Boston Women's Health Book Collective have enabled national women's health groups and networks to learn from each other and build solidarity in their search for solutions to the problems women define.

Regional coalitions like the Latin American and Caribbean Women's Health Network (LACWHN)[13] and the Asian and Pacific Women's Resource Collection Network have thousands of members in over 100 countries (Garcia-Moreno and Claro 1994). In some cases the members are themselves national networks representing dozens of local groups. In Latin America, the Chilean Open Forum for Reproductive Rights and Reproductive Health, founded in 1989, is an informal coalition of 45 women's groups and NGOs concerned with reproductive health; the Colombian Women's Network for Sexual and Reproductive Rights, formed in 1992 by 20 women's organizations, works on the decriminalization of abortion, sex education in schools, and a national women's health program that it helped formulate (Garcia-Moreno and Claro 1994).

The global women's health movement took shape from 1977 though international women and health meetings convened every three years.[14] European and North American women convened the first meeting, but the growing numbers of Southern women attending subsequent meetings pushed for a venue in the Southern hemisphere. These meetings have been particularly important in fostering debate on a wide variety of issues and in uniting the movement into a political force.

For many women's health movements around the world, the conferences held in Cairo in 1994 and Beijing in 1995, defined their agendas and directed them to work within the political system; many have seen the international forums as "windows of opportunity for policy advocacy" (Abdullah 2003, 35). The effectiveness of this strategy differs according to the goals that groups set for themselves. Although none of these movements focuses on a single issue, in several instances a single event or problem motivated their mobilization. Indian women reacted to the government's authoritarian population control efforts in the 1970s; Filipinas reacted to government policies in the 1980s and to pressure from the Roman Catholic hierarchy to restrict access to safe abortion and contraceptive choice.

The major preoccupation of the Moroccan women's movement is maternal mortality in the rural areas of the 14 poorest provinces in the country; assistance in childbirth and follow up are strikingly unequal compared to the urban centers. Sexually transmitted infections are a serious public health problem, especially as they increase women's vulnerability to AIDS. "Indeed, this situation is all the more alarming that social hypocrisy and the lack of power of women reinforce the fact women cannot protect themselves" (Association Démocratique des Femmes du Maroc 2003). The activism of conservative political groups opposed to governmental and nongovernmental sex education programs results in a low rate of condom use (under 6 percent). Although Morocco adopted the Cairo platform, the state still limits women's health concerns to reproductive matters. Only recently has the government recognized the concept of reproductive health, at least on paper. No data on breast and uterine cancer are available, and no specific program exists for these diseases. Nontherapeutic abortion is banned in Morocco yet thousands of women have abortions; poor women are at risk of damaging their health, if not endangering lives.

Women's priorities in Bosnia and Herzegovina reflect the problems of a war-torn country: rising domestic violence, forced labor, trafficking, disabilities, sexually transmitted infections, and a state medical system severely incapacitated by the war. Before the war primary health care was available free of charge. Now cantons can charge fees, even for abortion, which is legal. Before the war breast cancer was the leading cause of death among women. Now cervical cancer is a serious problem as clinics no longer conduct Pap tests regularly. Women's groups complain bitterly that even within the framework of human rights protection and analysis, the country's social, economic, and political interests, coupled with a tradition of bias, combine to cast women to the side as second-class citizens or persons of "special interest." Although many laws and statistics appear positive, or at least gender neutral, women's groups say that a deeper gender analysis leads to the overwhelming conclusion that women in Bosnia and Herzegovina have not yet attained any true measure of equality (NGOs in Bosnia and Herzegovina 2004).

In South Africa, the women's health movement is still demanding basics: sufficient nutritious food, clean water, adequate housing, sanitation, and safe waste disposal; all this against the legacy of apartheid, itself a violent system, which destroyed relationships and left in its wake an epidemic of violence against women and a tide of disabled people, not to mention the AIDS epidemic (Goosen and Klugman 1996). Contraceptive use and the legalization of abortion compete with memories of motherhood denied to African women. The government's inability to provide comprehensive reproductive health services has left women without the protection of Pap smears for early detection and cervical cancer the leading cause of women's cancer deaths in South Africa.

Women everywhere are fighting for control of decisions that affect their health. They are struggling with religious authorities who are raising issues about sex, sexuality, and gender. They argue with doctors, public health bureaucrats, medical and pharmaceutical companies, the health insurance industry, and religious leaders who are deciding what are the health issues within countries; they also debate with agencies like the United Nations Development Program (UNDP), the UN Population Fund (UNFPA), the United Nations Children's Fund (UNICEF), the U.S. Agency for International Development (USAID), the World Health Organization (WHO), and the World Bank, which are determining health policy at the international level. Some of these agencies are more receptive to women's advice than others, but as noted above, changing the language does not entail alteration of power structures. Women knew that rapid population growth was a problem deeply rooted in economic and social policies, and they argued convincingly that reproductive health services could not solve population problems. Yet some of the aid agencies still maintain that family planning is women's most important health care issue. Women recognized that violence against women was a health issue much earlier than any governmental or medical authorities did, but few governments implemented protective structures. Women saw that defining health care as a financial issue deprived the poor of services long before policymakers admitted the failure of the user-fee policy. And women understand that basic health services should be public, not private; that public policy determines who gets what kind of care while money governs access to the private sector; and that preventive services deserve priority over curative care.

Where women enter the discussion varies over time and from one group to another. When white middle class women started the debates about women's health in the United States, they could focus on doctor-patient relations and the desire for legal abortions. But for black women, the discussion has a much more basic starting point—with access to any health care (let alone its quality) and with the desire for healthy pregnancies and healthy children, which they felt was denied them because of sterilization abuse or because contraceptives were pushed on them—and they confront psychological hindrances like low self-esteem that grew out of poverty, unemployment, racism, and hassles with state agents like police and welfare workers. In international discussions, women in the global South also have to start the discussion with basics like the debt crisis; access to clean water, nutritious food, and adequate shelter; access to information and gainful work; access to basic health care and services for the prevention and treatment of AIDS; and an end to conflicts and wars (Stemerding 1997).

Women's achievements are fragile; they face new threats and old backlashes; their successes are reversible, even when legislators have made them the law of the land. Women have not yet achieved equality, not even in the most industrially advanced countries of the North.

CHAPTER TWO

The Global Context

North/South Inequities

Women's health movements exist in a global context of inequality between men and women, and between countries of the global North and South (formerly referred to as the First World and Third World). Inequality is an empirical concept measured in terms of income or consumption (usually a basic food basket) whereas equity is normative, a question of values associated with the idea of social justice. Economists generally derive definitions of poverty from measurements of inequality that are biased in favor of men. A broader measure of well-being that includes health is a more accurate definition of poverty for women excluded from the cash economy (Kabeer 1996). Economists generally define equity as the reduction of unfair and unjust differences (Gwatkin 2002).

Gender equality in health means that women and men have equal conditions for realizing their full rights and potential to be healthy, contribute to health development, and benefit from the results; gender inequity in health refers to those inequalities between women and men in health status, health care, and health work participation that are unjust, unnecessary, and avoidable. Gender equity strategies lead eventually to equality. Equity is the means, equality is the result (PAHO 2005).

Ill health and poverty are closely associated: in 2000 the World Health Organization (WHO 2000a) named poverty as a lethal cause of disease, but in a later report influenced by the World Bank, WHO calls disease a major determinant of poverty and makes investments to improve health a key strategy for economic development (Commission on

Macroeconomics and Health 2001). The link between poverty and ill health is interactive in that poverty shuts people out of health care and ill health reinforces poverty. An important difference distinguishes the two halves of the poverty-ill health equation. Naming poverty a cause of ill health emphasizes the social determinants of disease, such as class hierarchies, inequalities of income and wealth, and ethnic origin and racism; calling ill health a determinant of poverty diminishes the importance of health as a fundamental human right by focusing on economic productivity. Health is a fundamental human value, worthy of investment for its own sake; in becoming an instrument of development, health slips from consciousness, as does the vision of redistributing wealth as a worthy aim (Waitzkin 2003). Investment in health as a way to reduce poverty in poor countries enhances the economic prospects of the wealthy in both rich and poor countries. Poverty reduction projects per se do not contend with the dynamics of commercial markets that create poverty. The Women's Access to Health Campaign, which the Women's Global Network for Reproductive Rights and the People's Health Movement launched in 2003, argues that markets create conditions in which women's health and women's right to self-determination are sold (Hermans 2005).

Data demonstrate the close association of poverty with a shortened lifespan. An estimated 1.3 billion people, more than a quarter of those living in the global South, survive on less than one U.S. dollar a day (one definition of poverty), without any way to meet their basic needs, and they do not live beyond the age of 40. Despite many reports of improvement, in the decade of the 1990s, life expectancy at birth for over a billion people fell from 50 years to 40 years.

Inequality between classes is increasing within the United States, between the United States and other countries, and among countries divided along the North/South axis, as well as within all countries, North and South. High-income countries have 17 percent of the world's people and spend 89 percent of world expenditures on health services ($2.3 trillion) for 7 percent of the world's disease burden. (The United States accounts for about 40 percent of the global total.) In contrast low and middle-income countries have 83 percent of the world's population and account for 11 percent of world expenditures on health services ($0.3 trillion) for 93 percent of the world's disease burden. Health research is similarly skewed: 90 percent of annual funds spent worldwide are for diseases that affect 10 percent of the world's people; for example, of the 1,233 new medicines patented between 1975 and 1997, only 1 percent were for tropical diseases (Sharma 2000).

Two sets of data—on health services and health status—underscore these points. Combined public/private world expenditures in the health sector represented 9.3 percent of world GNP in 2000. Per person the worldwide average is $482 per year. People in high-income countries spend about $2,736 per person; in the United States that figure was $5,808 in 2003 (www.cms.hhs.gov accessed 7 February 2005). People in East Asia/Pacific, South Asia, and sub-Saharan Africa average $31 (World Bank 2003). Expenditures on pharmaceuticals are skewed: 74 percent of health expenditure in sub-Saharan Africa, 25 percent in Latin America and the Caribbean, and 7.4 percent in high-income countries is for medicines. In high-income countries, fewer than 40 percent of medicines are purchased privately, whereas the figure is 67 percent for sub-Saharan Africa and as high as 81 percent in Asia and the Pacific (PANOS 2002). People in high-income countries spend about $137.50 per person per year on pharmaceuticals; in sub-Saharan Africa, Latin America and the Caribbean, Asia and the Pacific Islands that figure was $15 per person per year in 1990 (Bennett, Quick, and Velasquez 1997).

Data on health status are similarly skewed. Average life expectancy at birth in the United States is 76 years; in sub-Saharan Africa it is 52 years and falling. Median age at death in the United States and Europe is 75 years; in Africa it is under 5 years (World Bank 1993). Economic inequalities between men and women persist: about 1.3 billion people live in absolute poverty, 70 percent of them women (UN 2000a). Women live longer than men as measured by life expectancy at birth, but during adolescence, women experience higher death rates than men in some countries because they bear children at too young an age. Women and girls also experience higher death rates in utero, infancy, and childhood in such countries as China and India where the preference for sons is strong.

North/South inequities are growing. As the richest nations get much richer and the poorest nations stagnate or grow even poorer, the divide between the poorest and richest countries widens. The data in table 2.1 are ranked according to GNP in 2003; for the poorest countries, the ranking is from lowest to highest incomes, whereas the richest countries are ranked in descending order.

The links between wealth and health, poverty and death are starkly visible on the global scale. Residents of Sierra Leone had an annual average income of $150 and could expect to live 37 years in 2003; residents of Luxembourg with an income of $39,840 could expect to live 78 years (www.worldbank.org accessed 1 August 2005). Some countries have a health status better than what their income rank would predict, for

Table 2.1 The poorest getting poorer, the richest getting (much) richer GNP per person (US$)

Poorest Countries	2003	1986	Richest Countries	2003	1986
Burundi	100	240	Norway	43,350	15,400
Congo (DRC)	100	160	Switzerland	39,880	17,680
Sierra Leone	150	310	USA	37,610	17,480
Malawi	170	160	Japan	34,510	12,840
Niger	200	260	Denmark	33,750	12,600
Mozambique	210	210	Sweden	28,840	13,160
Rwanda	220	290	U.K.	28,350	8,870
Nepal	240	150	Finland	27,010	12,160
Uganda	240	230	Austria	26,720	9,990
Central African Republic	260	290	Netherlands	26,310	10,020

Source: World Bank *World development report 2005*.

example Japan and Costa Rica; some have a lower than expected health status, for example the United States and South Africa. One explanation is that lower poverty rates and more egalitarian income distributions translate into longer life expectancy. Health benefits of higher incomes reach a point of diminishing returns around $15,000, suggesting that a transfer of income from the rich to the very poor would dramatically help extend the life expectancy of the very poor at little cost (in health terms) to the rich (Henwood 2000). Income explains more than 70 percent of the variation in world life expectancies.

National Health Inequalities

Societal averages like those given in national income data disguise as much as they reveal. The distribution of income within countries is central to an analysis of poverty and health. One measure of skewed income distribution is the Gini index: a score of 100 indicates perfect inequality; a score of 0 perfect equality. Table 2.2 gives a selection of highest and lowest scores; the highest are ranked in descending order and the lowest in ascending order. Remarkable are the number of wealthy countries with a low Gini index and the number of poor countries with a high Gini index. Unsurprising is the number of former socialist republics including parts of the former Yugoslavia that have low Gini indices.

Another source of data for inequity within countries is the percentage share of income or consumption by population quintiles. Distributional data by quintile refines the Gini index by showing how marginalized the poor are in unequal societies; and on the other side of the equation, income shares of the most equal countries show the degree to which the

Table 2.2 Gini indices for the 10 most unequal and 10 most equal countries

Country	Gini index >56	Country	Gini index <27
Namibia	70.7	Denmark	24.7
Lesotho	63.2	Japan	24.9
Botswana	63.0	Sweden	25.0
Sierra Leone	62.9	Belgium	25.0
Central African Republic	61.3	Czech Republic	25.4
South Africa	59.3	Slovak Republic	25.8
Brazil	59.1	Norway	25.8
Colombia	57.6	Bosnia & Herzegovina	26.2
Chile	57.1	Uzbekistan	26.8
Paraguay	56.8	Finland	26.9

Source: World Bank *World development report 2005*.

Table 2.3 Percentage share of income or consumption for 20 countries with lowest and highest percentiles for bottom and top 20 percent

Country	Lowest 20%	Highest 20%	Country	Lowest 20%	Highest 20%
Sierra Leone	1.1	63.4	Japan	10.6	35.7
Namibia	1.4	78.7	Czech Republic	10.3	35.9
Lesotho	1.5	66.5	Rwanda	9.7	39.1
South Africa	2.0	66.5	Finland	9.6	36.7
Central African Republic	2.0	65.0	Norway	9.6	37.2
Brazil	2.0	64.4	Bosnia and Herzegovina	9.5	35.8
Botswana	2.2	70.3	Uzbekistan	9.2	36.3
Paraguay	2.2	60.2	Slovenia	9.1	35.7
Panama	2.4	60.3	Sweden	9.1	36.6
Guatemala	2.6	64.1	Albania	9.1	37.4

Source: World Bank *World development report 2005*.

poor are included in society. Table 2.3 shows the lowest and highest quintiles of income shares: for the most unequal, countries are ranked by income share of lowest 20 percent in ascending order; and for the most equal, countries are ranked by income share of lowest 20 percent in descending order.

An understanding of health conditions that prevail in society as a whole does not necessarily elucidate the condition of different socioeconomic groups within society, especially that of the lowest or most disadvantaged groups. Although exclusive attention to the health of the disadvantaged focuses services to improve the health of the poor, it will do nothing to reduce differences between poor and rich. "For those oriented towards equality, the principal objective is the reduction of poor–rich health differences. Those concerned with health inequities are concerned with righting the injustice represented by inequalities or poor health conditions among the disadvantaged" (Gwatkin 2002, 4). A rare comparative study of child mortality in nine developing countries shows the largest difference between poor and nonpoor in Brazil (Wagstaff 2000). This finding conforms to the data in tables 2.2 and 2.3, which rank Brazil as a highly unequal society; Brazil's Gini index is 59.1 and the income share for the lowest quintile is 2.0 and for the highest 64.4. On the other hand, a low level of inequality in Pakistan did not protect against high rates of child mortality (Wagstaff 2000, 28). Unfortunately the child mortality survey does not differentiate between boys and girls.

One important question in examining inequities in health is what would constitute equitable distribution. Is it the same life expectancy for all individuals or the same health status at every stage of life (Gakidou, Murray, and Frenck 2000)? Or is it reduction in the consistent gaps between disadvantaged minorities and the majority? An extensive study of inequality in Great Britain revealed that with the National Health Service health improved throughout the population after the Second World War but that the gaps between social classes remained static (Townsend and Davidson 1982). A more recent study shows that the gap between the highest and lowest social classes widened in the latter part of the twentieth century (U.K. Office for National Statistics 2004). In the United States, the racial gap remains static—about twice as many black as white infants die each year and about four times as many black as white women die in pregnancy and childbirth—although the rates declined between 1900 and 2003.

Neither question addresses the inequities of poor women's health status relative to that of poor men.

Gender, Health, and Poverty

The WHO and World Bank studies of inequality cited above do not examine differences between women and men among the poor, just as they do not break down data for deaths of poor infants and children by sex. Mainstream health policy emphasizes women's special health needs less as a basic right and more as a cost effective means to improve child welfare. Typically, maternal and child health services overemphasize the synergy between the health of women and their children while overlooking nonreproductive health needs of poor women, as well as the broader range of gender-related factors that determine health status and care (Oxaal with Cook 1998).

This failure to value women lies at the core of women's health problems. Women's health movements pushed relentlessly for the collection of sex-disaggregated data that would reveal the subordinate position of women, the way gender roles shape women's health needs, and how the oppression of women acts to deprive them of needed health care. Collections of statistics and national data sets—the basis of social programs—still routinely fail to count women or disaggregate data by sex. Some societies attach no positive value to girls at birth, leading to infanticide and neglect in the early years, or even to avoidance of the birth of girls, resulting in high rates of abortion of female fetuses. In other societies, women are valuable only if, and for as long as, they can bear children: the status of infertile and post-menopausal women is low. Even when a society attaches importance to women bearing children, governments may not allocate resources to women's health care. This seems contradictory, but the effect can be seen in high mortality rates in pregnancy and childbirth.

Maternal death rates vary dramatically North and South, as shown in table 2.4. In industrial countries, maternal mortality averages 13 deaths per 100,000 live births, a 1 in 4,000 lifetime risk of dying from pregnancy; in sub-Saharan Africa that figure is 940 deaths per 100,000 live births, a 1 in 16 lifetime risk. In industrial countries, trained personnel attend 99 percent of births; in South Asia, only 35 percent of births are attended (UNICEF 2005).

Table 2.4   Maternal mortality ratios 2000. Adjusted rates and lifetime risk of maternal death

Poorest Countries	Rate	Risk 1 in:	Richest Countries	Rate	Risk 1 in:
Burundi	1,000	12	Norway	16	2,900
Congo (DRC)	990	13	Switzerland	7	7,900
Sierra Leone	2,000	6	USA	17	2,500
Malawi	1,800	7	Japan	10	6,000
Niger	1,600	7	Denmark	5	9,800
Mozambique	1,000	14	Sweden	2	29,800
Rwanda	1,400	10	U.K.	13	3,800
Nepal	740	24	Finland	6	8,200
Uganda	880	13	Austria	4	16,000
Central African Republic	1,100	15	Netherlands	16	3,500

Source: UNICEF *The state of the world's children 2005.*

Direct and indirect factors lead to poverty among women; some are a function of sex, some of gender, some a combination of both. Marriage is a social institution, a function of gender; childbearing is biological, a function of sex; in combination, early marriage and early childbearing can lead to poorer health and greater poverty. Most world regions show some improvement in the quality of women's lives, but early marriage and childbearing remain problematic: in 3 of 5 countries in Southern Asia and in 11 of 30 countries in sub-Saharan Africa, at least 30 percent of young women age 15 to 19 have been married (UN 2000a). In 19 countries (16 of them in sub-Saharan Africa) more than half of the women aged 25 to 29 had given birth before age 20 (Mensch, Bruce, and Greene 1998).

The health status of men and women at the same level of poverty is different because of differences in power, nutrition, work, and work hazards, which may be more important indicators of differences in well-being along gender lines than income-based measures that relate to only one aspect of poverty (Quisumbing, Haddad, and Peña 2001). Poverty and gender are also linked to mental illness, greater vulnerability to violence, and the stigma attached to certain health conditions (Oxaal with Cook 1998). In almost all countries, poor women have lower levels of education and fewer assets than men, indicators of massive discrimination against women who are denied access to and control of resources. It would therefore be quite remarkable if differences in the health status of men and women at the same level of poverty were not large.

As a consequence of their greater poverty, the priorities of women in the South are different from those of men; they are also different from the preoccupations and concerns of women in the North. These differences explain in part why women in the South feel the need to analyze global economic arrangements like trade agreements. To formulate a critique of the Beijing Platform for Action,[1] Indian women created a coordination unit and broadened consultations with women at the grassroots throughout the country (WGNRR 1995). The members of the unit objected to the apparent acceptance of a need to work within the boundaries created by the international order. They doubted whether socioeconomic systems, which structural adjustment programs shore up, stabilize, and make more unrelenting, could open up possibilities for the liberation of women. Structural adjustment programs push the majority of the poor to the margins, narrow their choices, and relegate women to the role of childbearing. To argue that markets are the answer to poverty, that poverty cannot be helped without economic growth while failing to question how the benefits of the market will reach those who

are not a part of it, is to overlook the issue of equity and the women who
bear the brunt of neoliberal economic policies. For the Indian coordination unit it was imperative to express health concerns as demands for
gainful work for all women and men. The women demanded a multi-
pronged attack on poverty, social injustice, and cultural myths, as well as
the identification of critical areas of health need for which the government should provide primary health care at basic, secondary, and tertiary
levels.

The Global Context of Women's Health Care

Poverty and subordinate gender roles constrain poor women and girls
making them the least likely to have access to appropriate care and to
seek adequate treatment. Household duties, work, and care giving consume their time, and the way households allocate resources and make
decisions conspire to limit women's access to health care. Additional
legal, social, and cultural factors hinder poor women seeking health care.
Gender affects health policy, financing, and service delivery; for example, maternal and child health services are generally part of public health
services that are chronically underfunded. Also, the decision to impose
user fees (patients' direct payment to health facilities) affects poor
women, who have little access to cash.

Women's groups are challenging international institutions that pro-
claim that poverty is women's number one health issue while developing policies that increase poverty in many countries. These women are
asking why funds are available for contraception but not for health care,
and why access to affordable, good-quality medicines and healthcare is
still a distant reality despite promises, usually in the form of unattained
goals like "Health for all by the year 2000."

The Health Impacts of International Institutions and Policies

Of primary concern is a broad array of neoliberal economic policies—
privatization, deregulation, and free trade—that negatively affect poor
women's health in multiple ways. The International Monetary Fund and
the World Bank, which dictate world health policy (a role formerly
assigned to WHO), impose these neoliberal economic policies on loan
recipients in the South. They have counseled privatization across the
board in industries as different as telecommunications and health care
with no regard for the inability of patients (as distinguished from consumers) to access information critical to decisions about their care.
Neoliberal health policies call for the commercialization of clinics,

hospitals, doctors' practice, and the distribution of drugs. Cutbacks in public health and the privatization of education result in the training of fewer doctors, nurses, and sanitarians. Budget reductions and the privatization of water supplies also affect environmental health conditions, raising the incidence of cholera and diarrheal diseases. The principle is that users must pay for services; the problem is that women rarely control cash and cannot pay. So, fewer women turn to trained personnel for assistance in childbirth and maternal death rates rise, especially in Africa.

Deregulation benefits multinational pharmaceutical companies by allowing them to set prices, control patents, and promote marketing practices that limit the number of people with access to drugs. The multinational pharmaceutical companies invest little in tropical disease research—there is still no vaccine for malaria, for example, and malaria kills over one million people every year, mainly African children.

Free trade is supposed to open up markets for agricultural products from the global South, but because agribusiness is selling genetically modified seeds and crops that many Northern countries reject, Africans and Asians cannot sell their produce. The large market for beef (for fast food hamburgers) means larger production of animal feed crops (as opposed to human food crops), often in countries short of arable land and water. Simultaneously, neoliberal policies dictate austerity budgets and reduced food subsidies, so the poor pay more for staples. Malnutrition and anemia are major problems of poor women and children in the global South, which food aid sometimes can alleviate, but some Northern countries use food aid as a weapon, as punishment and rewards for votes in the UN, for example.

Another group of neoliberal policies concerns population control, family planning, and abortion. The international organizations unanimously advocate and implement birth control policies, including UN agencies like the United Nations Population Fund (UNFPA) and large nongovernmental organizations funded by Northern governments like the U.S.-based Family Health International. World Bank policies put population control as the number one priority in social aid programs. Women (and very rarely men) are the targets of these programs, which aim to reduce population growth by limiting births (they pay less attention to migration and death, the other dimensions of population dynamics that also influence population numbers). Quotas for contraceptive use lead to abusive, coercive practices in countries like Indonesia, and sterilization camps in India and more recently Peru (see chapter 6 for a full discussion of reproductive rights).

Yet another group of policies concerns the AIDS pandemic. At issue is the dominant medical approach to controlling the spread of HIV, which combines testing and condom use with behavioral change; more recently these programs have included palliative drug treatment. The Bush administration promotes a more limited "abstinence only" education program that emphasizes counseling as the answer to the AIDS epidemic, even though WHO and other international agencies believe it is ineffective. The Clinton administration, which resisted the introduction of antiretroviral drugs in Africa, backed the pharmaceutical industry's lawsuit against South Africa to keep that country from producing or importing generic versions of antiretrovirals. Under pressure from the South African Treatment Advisory Campaign (TAC) and negative world press, the industry eventually withdrew the lawsuit; but the Bush Administration is reluctant to authorize purchases of generic antiretroviral drugs through its aid programs.

International Trade Agreements and Women's Access to Healthcare

A specific aspect of neoliberal policies very damaging to health is the regulation of global commerce. International trade agreements are one of several economic arrangements that negatively affect women's health, and the World Trade Organization (WTO)[2] is one of the institutions that impose detrimental policies. On the occasion of the 15th international day of action for women's health on 28 May 2002, the Women's Global Network for Reproductive Rights joined the People's Health Assembly to issue a call for action on international trade agreements that threaten women's access to healthcare (WGNRR 2002a). Although the specialized agencies of the United Nations claim to be working to reduce poverty and improve women's lives, the international community led by the G8 nations[3] is creating institutions that undermine the provision of the goods and services women need to survive. Two such agreements, TRIPS (Trade-Related Aspects of Intellectual Property Rights) and GATS (General Agreement on Trade in Services), affect women negatively in three ways: by curtailing access, they affect women as users of health care systems and of medicines; by trading and privatizing services, they affect women as providers of care; and by patenting medicinal plants, they affect women as cultivators of these herbs.

TRIPS is an agreement reached by members of the WTO with respect to pharmaceutical products whereby it protects the development of new medicines. The agreement has the effect of raising drug prices, with severe consequences for the poor. Drugs can account for as much as 40 percent of health budgets in poor countries where doctors are scarce

and auxiliary staff use drugs to treat millio⌐
As drug prices rise, however, the number o.
shrinks.

Because so few developing countries have ⌐
ufacture pharmaceuticals, WTO allows for importa.
pulsory license, waiving TRIPS arrangements; com⌐
override patents in return for payment of royalties. Fu
urges developed country members to promote the transfer ⌐
ogy and capacity building in the pharmaceutical sector and to ⌐
technical cooperation (WTO 2003). But in practice corporations
not agreed to such waivers or transfers of technology. ACTUP (ALL
Coalition to Unleash Power) and the South African Treatment
Advisory Campaign (TAC) initiated a broad international campaign to
make antiretroviral drugs available in Africa, forcing the WTO to
loosen the TRIPS agreement adopted at its 2001 meeting in Doha
(WTO 2001). The new agreement gives each member the right to
waive patent protections by granting manufacturing licenses under
exceptional circumstances. It also frees members to determine what
constitutes circumstances of extreme urgency or a national emergency;
for example, public health crises, including those relating to tuberculosis, malaria, and AIDS, can represent a national emergency or
circumstance of extreme urgency.

GATS is a set of multilateral rules governing international trade in
services (for example, telecommunications, banking, accountancy, and
travel). Developed in response to the huge growth of the service economy over the past 30 years, and the greater potential for trading services
brought about by the communications revolution, GATS gives members the right to regulate the supply of services in pursuit of national policy objectives and the right to specify which services they wish to open
to foreign suppliers and under what conditions. WTO says the guidelines are sensitive to public policy concerns in important sectors such as
health care, public education, and cultural industries in the developing
and least-developed countries. The overarching principle, according to
the WTO, is one of flexibility, while stressing the importance of liberalization in general and ensuring foreign service providers have effective
access to domestic markets (www.wto.org accessed 5 August 2005).
Critics of GATS point out that the real principle is public subsidies for
the private sector, which they see in the proposal of guaranteed funding
for private providers, including those that are profit making (Waitzkin
2003). For instance, the ability of multinational corporations to sell
publicly funded health services has emerged in GATS.

Women's Health Movements

Two-Way Interaction between Women
in the Global North and South

liberal economic philosophy, which originated in the North, profits
ltinational corporations based in Northern countries. Structural
justment and trade agreements are but two examples of Northern
eoliberal policies that affect women in the South. A range of national
policies touches women North and South. How women's movements
respond to them has a direct bearing on women's health. This is a two-
way street.

Two questions in the global context of women's activism are: how
does the status of women in the South affect women in the North, and
how do decisions taken in the North affect women in the South? In
principle, activists from nations in the North will contest the policies of
their governments so that women in the South can advance their own
causes in their respective countries; together coalitions of women North
and South can confront the international agencies. Some issues seem to
pit the interests of women in the South against those of women in the
North, however; others appear to have a similarly negative effect on
women everywhere.

The status of women in the South affects women in the North in several ways. One is the way low status and concomitant low wages drive
women out of the South to search for jobs that will support their families. Many end up as domestic and childcare workers for (relatively)
wealthy women in the North. In what Hochschild (2000) calls "the
nanny chain," migrant workers must find other women to care for their
own children left behind, part of an economy of care aggravated by the
decision to privatize social services in the North.

A second way in which the status of women in the South links to the
lives of women in the North is through foreign adoptions and surrogacy
arrangements. Some critics call this the rental of wombs and ponder the
ethical implications of declining fertility in the North creating a demand
for children from the South. In India (and other countries), foreigners'
demand for children to adopt has led to baby trafficking (Bonner 2003a).
Gita Ramaswamy, a long-time union organizer in India, is demanding a
nationwide moratorium on foreign adoptions for several years, arguing
that poverty and the degradation of women in Indian society induce
many poor women to sell their baby girls. The Indian government
allows foreigners to adopt babies as a stopgap solution rather than address
the problems. What drives baby trafficking is the demand; offers of what
to poor women are irresistible amounts of money persuade them to sell

their babies. A mother with four girls sold h
earns 60 cents a day and her husband earns $1
(not their own). The buyer, a woman from ano.
baby (and 19 others from the same village) to some
the children ended up in orphanages that offered then.
foreign couples (Bonner 2003b).

The global "gag rule" prohibits programs receiving U..
providing or promoting abortion, from advocating change in th
governmental policies of any foreign country concerning abortic
even mentioning abortion as an option when counseling pregn.
women (WGNRR 2000c, 20; Rayman-Read 2001). Women's groups
struggle around the global gag rule, which vividly illustrates the impact
of decisions taken in the North on women in the South. The administration of President Ronald Reagan adopted the rule as a response to
allegations by conservatives opposed to the termination of pregnancy
about the connection between UN funds and coercive abortion policies
in China.[4] In July 2002, the administration of G.W. Bush withheld
$34 million for family planning programs in all countries through
UNFPA. Fact-finding missions from the United States and Great Britain
have investigated the allegations and found no evidence of a link
between the UN family planning fund and abortion or forced sterilization in China. UNFPA funds are not used to promote or fund abortions
as a method of family planning in any country; in fact through a pilot
program UNFPA has persuaded government officials in China to end
coercive family planning policies, part of China's "one family, one
child" population control policy, in 32 Chinese counties. The effect of
the gag rule is to reduce access to contraceptives, which seems to contradict the overall international plan to reduce population growth. The
U.S. decision to withhold funds affects many countries that receive aid
from UNFPA, which estimates the loss of funding will lead to some two
million unintended pregnancies, nearly 800,000 abortions, and 4,700
maternal deaths.

The global gag rule also affects the work of health care for women in
clinics that do not provide abortions because groups that depend on
United States Agency for International Development (USAID) funding
are afraid to treat women suffering the effects of septic abortions or give
post-abortion contraceptive counseling. The logic seems to be that a
woman who dies of septic abortion cannot repeat her mistake, and her
death will discourage others from following her example. When Susana
Galdos Silva, cofounder of Movimiento Manuela Ramos, a Peruvian
women's health group that receives family planning funds from USAID,

...d to testify before the Senate Foreign Relations Committee in July she had to request explicit prior authorization from a U.S. court. ...n one level, policies like the global gag rule aggravate the problems ...oor women who give birth to more children than they want. On a ...cond level, such policies are a part of the struggles of women in the North to preserve their right to abortion. On a third level, because illegal abortions account for 13 percent of maternal deaths globally and women with septic abortions can occupy 50 percent of hospital beds, debates about abortion in the North directly affect women's health generally in the global South.

The practice of using foreign aid to manipulate national family planning programs has a long history. International agencies have stipulated that countries must have population control programs to receive foreign aid and loans, a requirement that can lead to mass sterilization and the imposition of family planning quotas that force women to accept contraception. The U.S. government has used foreign aid programs to dump contraceptives banned in the United States; for example, it shipped overseas copper T intrauterine devices long after the government banned their sale in U.S. markets. Women's groups campaigned successfully to stop such practices.

From the perspective of women in the South, advocates of human development from the North merge health issues into universal reproductive health and rights issues instead of visualizing health issues as women of different regions see them (Qadeer 1998). The problem with this sort of universalizing is that reproductive health does not have the same meaning for all women, as white women organizing for the liberalization of abortion laws in the North discovered when women of color complained that their first concern was sterilization abuse, not access to abortion. Many oppressed women find they must claim the right to motherhood when faced with coercive birth control programs.

In some instances, women North and South are common victims of programs, for example, the use of new technology. Agribusiness, which includes multinational food corporations, controls food supplies all over the world, affecting obesity in the North and undernutrition in the South by their choice of production and distribution techniques.

Sex selection technology (the use of ultrasound and amniocentesis to detect the sex of the fetus) has played into the hands of patriarchs in societies that prefer sons to daughters. Whom should women hold accountable for the estimated 100 million missing women (Dugger 2001)? (See chapter 6 for an extended discussion of this issue.)

Economic, Social, and Political
Determinants of Health

The final section of this chapter shifts the discussion from economic to sociological theory. My study of colonial medicine in East Africa revealed the mismatch between medical services designed in the metropolitan centers and transferred to their possessions and the health conditions that colonial economic policies created in their empires (Turshen 1975). Tracing the development of the medical-industrial complex in Great Britain, my study exposed the narrow theoretical basis of biomedical services that used hospitals as the primary venue for treatment. This curative model of care was particularly unsuited to sparsely populated agrarian societies subjected to forced labor drafts in mines and on plantations.

Social and community medicine today takes for granted the roles of economics, society, and politics in the health status of people and in their access to health care. Yet this is still not the dominant view in clinical medicine or even in public health. Other theories of disease, singly or in eclectic combination, still determine much of our understanding of ill health and dictate the solutions that are developed and applied. Theories of disease causation (etiologies) carry a philosophy and an ideological conviction with political consequences attached to them. They condition the direction of medical research, in part by controlling public health policy and the grant-making process. Most practitioners of medicine and public health are pragmatists, not theoretical purists, and they select whatever response seems useful in a particular situation; not all are aware of or interested in the distant determinants of disease, the ideological implications of their diagnosis, or the economic, social, or political consequences of their treatment decisions.

When the germ theory of disease became prominent in the biological era of the late nineteenth century, economic, social, and political determinants of health that had been of interest to pioneers like Johann Peter Frank (1745–1821) and Rudolf Virchow (1821–1902) fell out of favor. Germ theory holds that every illness has a specific cause (microbial or viral; for example, the tubercle bacillus causes tuberculosis) and every illness (theoretically) has a specific prevention (BCG vaccine) and cure (surgery or drugs like PAS, INH, and rifampicin). This theory was useful in explaining contagious disease in the late nineteenth century and used to good effect in controlling bacterial diseases like typhoid and diphtheria. Germ theory operates in the biological realm, outside of economic, social, and political factors. It does not explain why only some people who harbor the germ fall ill and why death rates vary among those who fall ill. Germ theory looks for the magic bullet, the one-shot cure or prevention. This approach dominated cancer research for decades, deflecting attention from environmental causes of disease. The model for the germ theory is the global public health campaign that wiped out smallpox. The use of a freeze-dried vaccine resulted in the elimination of this disease, but such campaigns rarely change people's living and working conditions.

Genetics, the study of heredity, another development in elucidating disease etiology, dates to the late nineteenth century. Medical genetics traces disorders to genetic abnormalities, either inherited or resulting from mutations. The field has had a checkered history because eugenicists and sociobiologists have misused the theory and have used genetics to justify racial oppression. The eugenics movement was dedicated to improving the human species through the crude use of birth control to affect hereditary factors (see chapter 6 on women's reproductive rights for a discussion of eugenics and sterilization). Sociobiology, the study of the biological origins of animal and human behavior, is the theory that behavior is genetically determined. Spearheaded by E.O. Wilson's *Sociobiology: the new synthesis* published in 1975 and Richard Dawkins's *The selfish gene* published in 1976, the theory gave eugenics a new disguise. Progressive scientists like Jon Beckwith exposed sociobiology's links to genetic determinism, eugenics, racism, and National Socialism and also noted the field's crude sexism. Despite its disrepute, sociobiology survives as evolutionary biology, "a grab bag of genetic determinism, biologized philosophy and old-fashioned racism and sexism" (Marks 2003, 30).

Gene theory has achieved new prominence in these conservative times with the human genome project and advances in microbiology. But genetics alone explains only 5 percent of disease; it does not explain the other 95 percent. Genetics rests solidly in the realm of biology, and economic, social, and political factors seem to be irrelevant. Applied gene theory uses genetic engineering, fetal surgery, genetic screening, and counseling to affect disease. Gene theory is applied in the workplace to exclude those workers determined by management to be genetically susceptible to certain diseases; this strategy obviates the need to alter the workplace environment, making it safe for all workers.

By the 1930s, chronic diseases were overtaking communicable diseases as leading causes of death in the North. It was soon clear that neither germ theory nor gene theory could explain these conditions or offer much in the way of treatment. A new theory emerged, multifactorial causation, meaning that more than one cause is involved in disease, that race, economic status, cultural values, and social conditions may all play a role. Multifactorial causation explains that most diseases, especially chronic conditions, have many causes; for example, most physicians now acknowledge that any or all of the following factors—genetics, diet, behavior, smoking, exercise, and stress—cause heart disease. This theory represents the first time since the biological era that medical researchers have taken social factors into consideration in understanding disease etiology. Multifactorial causation opened the way to multiple interventions; for example, in heart disease, doctors could select from an array of solutions—surgery, pacemakers, drugs to control blood pressure and cholesterol, low-fat diets, exercise regimens, stress management, biofeedback, meditation, and so on.

Multifactorial theory does not tell us whether the associations are causal or statistical correlations (like smoking and lung cancer), nor does it tell us the direction of the causation (does smoking kill workers or does working kill smokers?). It does not tell us which factor to look at in the first place; whatever we select to examine reflects our biases and ideology. Male researchers routinely overlook factors that are significant in women's lives and thereby miss the different symptoms of, for example, heart disease in women. Multifactorial analyses deconstruct societies into quantifiable components or aggregate individual risk factor frequencies into a "social analysis": this is positivist scientific reasoning, based on the belief that if one observes, describes, quantifies, and explains all the components of a system, one can generate an objectively real understanding of it (Decosas 2002). But populations are not systems and positivist causal reasoning does not help uncover human disease etiologies.

Because the recommended alterations in behavior are individual and not society-wide, the changes are minimal and short-lived. The emphasis on behavioral change led some researchers to analyze the role of lifestyles in disease. This theory, which became popular in the 1960s, claims that one's behavior (eating, drinking, smoking, exercise, sexual activity) determines one's health. Behavioral scientists often apply lifestyle analyses to disadvantaged cultural groups to explain their disease patterns. The theory singles out individuals and links behavioral change to belief in individual responsibility for personal health. It is a narrower etiological explanation than multifactorial causation because it focuses almost exclusively on social factors. Lifestyle theory relies on behavioral change through legal restraints (for example, legislating the use of helmets and seat belts) or education, persuasion, and coercion. Lifestyle theorists believe in human agency, free will, and freedom of choice, as well as individual responsibility. The theory leads to victim blaming and to the abdication of societal responsibility. It ignores the economic and political determinants of people's health.

In the 1970s and 1980s, progressive social scientists and health workers around the world, dissatisfied with the medical models of disease, began the work of reinterpreting disease history. The forerunners were some avant-guard revolutionists in France at the end of the eighteenth century; the nineteenth century contributions of two German scientists, Johann Peter Frank and Rudolf Virchow, mentioned above; early experiments with public health in the Soviet Union; an experimental primary care service unit in, Pholela, a local community in the Drakensberg mountains of Natal, South Africa, set up by Sydney and Emily Kark in 1940; the Canadian physician, Norman Bethune, who worked among the tubercular poor in Montreal and then went to China; Georges Canguilhem whose 1943 medical thesis, *The Normal and the Pathological*, exposed the theoretical lapses of mechanical explanations of diabetes; Joshua Horn working in the People's Republic of China shortly after the 1949 revolution and reporting on the remarkable advances in public health; and René Dubos's rethinking of the ecology of disease. From the 1950s the hearings held in the U.S. Congress by Senator Estes Kefauver revealed unconscionable practices by the pharmaceutical industry; and 1960s activists like those at the New York-based Health Policy Advisory Center (HealthPAC) and journalists like Morton Mintz (1965) published muckraking exposés of drug companies. Consumer groups organized around issues in the global South like the unethical sales of infant formula to mothers who could afford neither the powder, nor clean water, nor sterilized bottles in which to feed it to their infants (INFACT, church groups, Baby Foods Action Group).

A North American group, with links to European, Latin American, Asian, and African scholars and a background in Marxist scholarship and New Left activism, met regularly in the 1980s to develop what we came to call the social production of health and disease, a theory that broad economic, social, and political systems produce health and illness. This theory differs from multifactorial causation, which categorizes populations according to factors like race, sex, education, and income and computes their relative influence statistically; multifactorial causation does not explain the significance of the factors or how they might relate to one another. Social production theory has an overarching explanation of the dynamics behind the factors—it is not race that explains black/white differences in mortality and morbidity, it is racism; it is not sex that explains male/female differences, it is sexism. Income is not a parallel characteristic; it is a proxy for inequality. Social production theory points out that prejudice, discrimination, and racism are characteristics of social systems, whereas race, sex, education, and income are characteristics that sociologists use to classify individuals. Social organization produces health or disease through equal or unequal distribution of income and wealth among social classes, genders, races, and ethnicities, both within countries and globally.

Health differences between women and men within any given socioeconomic group (whether of class, caste, or race) can be significant. The patterns of tuberculosis infection and illness vary between poor women and men, as do those for coronary heart disease between richer women and men. Various studies of inequalities in health have shown that although class is the main determinant of health inequalities, significant differences in health outcomes by race and gender remain within each class level. These differences may not be uniform or even move in the same direction. Although health research largely confirms the expected differences between the polar extremes of the social gradient, that is, between rich, white men on the one hand, and poor women of color on the other, no obvious or linear pattern emerges as one moves along the social gradient. In the United States for example, welfare policies have targeted poor women with dependent children. In the absence of general unemployment benefits, this has led to worse health access for poor men than for poor women. It is precisely because of these complex and nonlinear patterns that health research and policy need to pay them greater attention (Sen, George, and Östlin 2002).

Consequences of Poverty and Sexism for Women's Health Care

The theory that health and disease are socially produced has especial relevance for women's health. It moves the critique of women's medical care out of biological and behavioral realms into analyses of economic, social, and political determinants. It has given women's health movements a theoretical basis for their demands by providing an explanation of overlapping factors, and it has enabled women to analyze the intersection of multiple conditions like poverty, sexism, and racism.

Poverty is central to women's experience of motherhood and to whether women survive pregnancy and childbirth. Decisions about how many children to have and when to have them are family decisions, not individual choices, in many communities. The decision to seek trained help when complications arise is not a woman's to take, and in any case she would rarely have her own money to pay the bill at a clinic, pharmacy, or hospital. Nor does she have the information to estimate the seriousness of her situation, as she is often illiterate. Lack of income and lack of education are related reflections of her dependent status. Unequal power relations reverberate through her life, dictating marriage (including polygamy), childbearing, and work. To introduce biomedical obstetric technology into this situation can lead to the consolidation of power relations in which women are the losers (De Koninck 1998).

The health effects of poverty are apparent in women working too many hours each day, working in hazardous conditions, and eating too little food or food of poor quality. Other health effects are apparent in women's poor mental health, their vulnerability to violence, and the stigma they suffer due to certain health problems. Poor nutrition is key to long-term health effects: gender inequality and poverty combine to produce ill health for women and girls, and ongoing poverty means that the ill effects of undernourishment and overwork, especially during pregnancy or lactation, will carry over to the next generation. Some kinds of ill health—for example, the parasitic diseases leishmaniasis, schistosmiasis, lymphatic filariasis, and onchocerciasis, which cause profound incapacity and disfigurement—may lead to the social exclusion of women, deepening their poverty and creating a cycle of ill health and poverty (Oxaal with Cook 1998).

The Compound Impact of Racism

For women of color, problems of racial discrimination compound gender stereotypes resulting in gendered racial stereotypes. In Great Britain, researchers observed that within the National Health Services, health workers assume that Afro-Caribbean women are feckless and irresponsible, while Asian women are compliant but stupid, that West Indian women have no culture, whereas culture is the problem for Asian women (Kushnick, quoted in Geiger 2002). A particularly damaging experience is the assumption that every individual of the group shares the same characteristics, regardless of age, education, income, and occupation. The classic example is the emergency room clinician who assumes that the middle-class professional African American woman he is examining is an unemployed welfare recipient (Gamble, quoted in Geiger 2002).

Racial and ethnic differentials persist in maternal and infant mortality rates, with indigenous women in some countries experiencing higher maternal mortality than women of other groups. Indigenous women in Peru experience maternal mortality rates twice as high as the general population. The average infant mortality rate of 80 per 1,000 live births in Guatemala jumps to 160 per 1,000 in the highland Indian areas. The UN Special Rapporteur on violence against women in the report on her mission to South Africa noted that while maternal mortality is 2.6 per 100,000 births for black women, it is only .003 per 100,000 births for white women (Coomaraswamy 2001). Throughout U.S. history, the health status of people of color—African Americans, Native Americans, Latinos, and several Asian subgroups—has never equaled or even approximated that of white Americans. Although the health of the whole population has improved, people of color still experience more illness and die earlier. In 1995, the overall African American death rate was 60 percent higher than that of whites, the same disparity found in 1950 (Geiger 2002). Latinas in the United States are twice as likely as white women to die in childbirth, and African American women are four times as likely as whites to die. Psychiatrists diagnose African Americans as psychotic more often than whites but they give African Americans antipsychotic medications less often. Doctors are also more likely to hospitalize African Americans involuntarily, to regard them as potentially violent, and to place them in restraints or in isolation. Over the past 20 years in the United States, infection with HIV and clinical progression to AIDS have disproportionately affected African Americans and Latinos and are now among the leading causes of death for these groups. The overall pattern of racial and ethnic discrimination is clear: African Americans and Latinos are less likely than whites to receive a variety of medications or to undergo some diagnostic procedures (Geiger 2002). Reviews of the literature find these differences between the treatment of whites and blacks at every age level and in both outpatient and inpatient services (Geiger 2002). A review of more than 150 studies shows that among the multiple causes of racial and ethnic disparities in health care in the United States, provider and institutional bias are significant contributors (Geiger 2002).

Traditional public health analyses attribute disparities in health status to socioeconomic status (low income, lack of education, unemployment), lack of access to health care, lifestyle choices, behavioral risks, job hazards, environmental dangers, poor housing, poor nutrition, and cultural beliefs about health and illness that are inimical to good health and health care. These analyses explain the disparities in terms of biological and genetic differences, despite repeated proofs that race is a social construction, not a biological concept. Public health analysts rarely acknowledge the contribution of class combined with the lifelong experiences of racial and ethnic discrimination: the historic and persistent disadvantages that oppress people of color in social structures.

Four North/South comparisons emerge from the data: 1) the image of the largely rich, white global North and its photographic negative in the largely poor, nonwhite South (the gross inequalities are described above in the section on "North/South inequities"), 2) the correspondences between the status of women in the South and that of women in the North, 3) the parallels between disadvantaged groups in the South and those in the North—an issue discussed at the United Nations World Conference Against Racism, Racial Discrimination, Xenophobia and Related Intolerance in 2001, and 4) the similarities and differences between groups of women of color in the North and in the South. These comparisons go beyond North/South, rich/poor, black/nonblack, and male/female binaries; they lead to the analytical conundrum of computing the cumulative corrosive effects of multiple inequalities and prejudices on health.

The Intersection of Sexism, Racism, and Economic Inequality

Identity politics often redefines our multidimensional selves with a single feature, deflecting our attention from inequalities and inequities. Rejecting that narrow approach, women's movements are looking more closely at the interactions of sexism, racism, and economic inequality. Using the awkward term intersectionality, women are trying to describe the crossroads, interweavings, and layers of our lives.

Sen, George, and Östlin (2002) observe that researchers usually define gender as a set of social roles but do not use roles to define race or class dynamics, testifying to a tendency in policy circles to treat gender in isolation from structural analyses of inequality. An exclusive or excessive emphasis on roles leads to a focus on behavior change at the individual level, rather than on policy change at the societal level. In the health field, role analysis deflects our attention from gender as a distinct and powerful form of stratification that interacts with other social markers like class, race, ethnicity, and sexual orientation.

Although gross data exist for North/South differences and male/female differences, the data on racial, ethnic, and religious numerical minorities within countries of the South are largely nonexistent. In an issue of the *Bulletin of the World Health Organization* devoted to the theme of inequality and health, an article on child mortality observes "there has been no systematic examination of ethnic inequality in child survival chances across countries in the [sub-Saharan African] region" (Brockerhoff and

Hewitt 2000, 30). Geographical location of ethnic groups (residence in the largest city), household economic conditions, educational attainment, and nutritional status of the mothers, use of modern maternal and child health services including immunization, and patterns of fertility and migration were the criteria for determining inequality. The authors report no breakdown by sex. Racism, sexism, class prejudice, and discrimination—as either the legacy of colonial rule or the result of power struggles—were not issues considered relevant to inequality.

In nineteenth-century arguments about North/South hierarchies, authors invoked climatic advantages in the North to explain the superiority of its people; today economic disadvantage (sometimes socioeconomic disadvantage) is the common explanation of North/South mortality differentials. Both accounts let organizers, participants, and perpetuators of discriminatory institutions and systems of prejudice off the hook. Caste systems in India clearly affect people's life chances, yet few data quantify the impact of caste on health. Dalit women suffer from significantly lower levels of literacy than the general Indian population: 76 percent of Dalit women are illiterate compared with 49 percent of the total Indian population, and 83 percent of Dalit women drop out of secondary school. Researchers tend to use economic arguments like pressure to earn an income in poor households to explain this discrepancy (Women's Net accessed 26 June 2006). Although statistical offices have documented the association of high levels of income inequality and poor health, they have not explained the uneven experiences of minority communities that do not have the same rates of sickness and death. Societies privilege some minorities like whites in Namibia. Social cohesion mitigates risk in other minority communities; cohesion may come with an identifiable community leader or spokesperson, a newspaper in the community's language, and organizations that give a collective voice to the community and lead to collective action. But it is not enough to trace disparities in health status to disparate treatment, or to show the different outcomes that result from the minimal and delayed care of disadvantaged minorities when we control for socioeconomic status and access to health care. Intersectionality promises a much richer and deeper understanding of women's health.

Food Insecurity

This section on food insecurity concludes the chapter on the global context of women's health movements. Globalization integrates international markets for goods and services more closely than in the past; it also raises cross-border investment in production of goods and services. Above all, it creates the international governance frameworks and policies that seek to sustain both trends. As a result, globalization affects the availability of food and the quality of diets, in both the North and the South. Not coincidentally, food is the focus of widespread protest and the issue around which women have been organizing for decades. The effects of globalization have given a new impetus and urgency to these movements.

Biological differences between women and men complicate the analysis of discrimination against women in the field of health. Within health sciences, biology has greater influence on male/female differences than do wealth, income, caste, class, ethnicity, and race. But biology cannot fully explain women's health status or health care. Social determinants of health exacerbate biological vulnerabilities, and social disadvantages are prime determinants of inequitable health outcomes. Gender analyses allow researchers to distinguish and comprehend the social basis of differences between women and men and make it possible to dig beneath obvious biological difference to the deeper social bases of power and inequality (Sen, George, and Östlin 2002).

Malnutrition illustrates the complex interaction of biology and bias. Undernourished and malnourished people living in difficult conditions easily contract infectious diseases, and malnutrition magnifies the outcome of infection. Smallpox is one of the few infections in which the nutritional status of the host does not affect the outcome of the illness. The best-known synergy is between measles and malnutrition, sometimes a consequence of diarrheal disease, in young children. Despite decades of research on this synergy, studies do not routinely disaggregate data by sex in order to look at the contribution of sexism. Does the synergy affect girls more than boys? Organizations like WHO seem unable to coordinate the research of their women's health unit, which carries out gender analyses, with units studying nutrition or tropical diseases. Although health scientists know that malnutrition is the biggest risk factor in disease worldwide, households and health care facilities often fail to recognize the different nutritional needs of girls and women. Biases against girls and women are widely institutionalized. Economic differentials in property and inheritance, as well as divisions of labor within households and communities, reproduce those biases.

Nutritional deficiencies like iron-deficiency anemia and iodine deficiency affect maternal and child death rates as well as cognitive and physical development of children and the work productivity of adults (McNeil 2006; WHO 2004). Nearly 50 percent of women in developing countries suffer from anemia, which is probably the most common health problem affecting almost half of women of all ages in the global South (Paolisso and Leslie 1995). Anemic women who become pregnant may easily develop pregnancy complications.

Women have been in the forefront of demonstrations against rising prices of staple foods and the removal of government subsidies, a measure mandated by the World Bank as part of its structural economic reforms. In Khartoum, the capital city of Sudan, the Sudanese Feminist Union (1996) organized a large demonstration in 1979 to protest against the hike in the price of sugar. When police intervened, officers had to lead the charge because patrolmen refused to attack, saying they were convinced of the fairness of the women's demands for lower prices. Incidents like this one take place repeatedly all over the world. One study in Argentina collected reports on 289 "food riot episodes" occurring in December 2001: typical is a story from the city of Tucumán, where 150 women, who heard that the government was giving out food, walked to a municipal center; when nobody showed up to help them, they marched to a chain supermarket where rumor had it a food distribution was to take place. "As soon as they arrived, police fired rubber bullets and tear gas at the crowd. 'The government lied to us,' they said afterward, 'we came to ask for food and they held us back as if we were criminals'" (Auyero and Moran 2007, 17).

Worldwide, women are resisting the policies that destroy the basis of their livelihoods and food sovereignty. They are also creating alternatives to guarantee food security for their communities based on principles and methods different from those governing the dominant, profit-oriented global economy. Among the alternatives are localization and regionalization, nonviolence, equality and reciprocity, respect for the integrity of nature, understanding that humans are part of nature, and protection of biodiversity in production and consumption. Among the outstanding women leaders of the movements for food security are Vandana Shiva and Maria Mies. At the NGO meeting that preceded the Food and Agriculture Organization (FAO) conference on plant genetic resources in Leipzig, Germany, in June 1996,[5] Mies and Shiva, observing that the discussion on food security did not take into account women's worldwide provision of food to their families and communities, prepared the Leipzig Appeal.[6] Using a women's perspective the appeal rejected the trend to remove food security from the hand of communities and farmers; criticized neoliberal policies of global food trade and the genetic manipulation of food for the sake of profit; and critiqued the proposed policy of globalization, liberalization, and industrialization of food production, trade, and consumption.

In a continuation and extension of industrialization and the worldwide trade of food, the cheapest labor produces food where environmental protection is weakest. The market forces poor communities to produce luxury products for export to rich countries and classes to devastating effect: the disappearance of small farmers, the end of food self-sufficiency, reliance on monoculture, genetic manipulation of food, loss of biodiversity, and ecological unsustainability. FAO proposes this world agriculture policy, which causes poverty and malnutrition and displaces impoverished rural people who end up as marginal members of society in overcrowded megacities without work, hope, or food, as a remedy for these very ills. The policies most affect poor rural women and children, the most vulnerable groups.

In Peru, Chile, and other countries of the South, women are fighting against this monopolistic policy, building their own communal food and health systems. Women in indigenous societies fight against land alienation, and women in export-oriented agriculture oppose hazardous chemicals. In the North, women who support them are calling for boycotts of such luxury export products as flowers, vegetables, and shrimp. Many groups in the North and South reject genetic manipulation of food, which industry presents as biotechnology necessary to feed a growing world population; however, animals in industrial farming systems consume 60 percent of cereals, leaving less and less land in the South for nourishing local people.

CHAPTER THREE

The Triple Day: Women's Home, Community, and Workplace Environments

This chapter considers women in their environments—their homes, their communities, and their workplaces. The term environment has several meanings here: it indicates physical, inorganic factors (soil, climate), biological factors (plants, animals, germs), and social factors (human activity—everything from the built environment to human behavior). Many studies document the mutual interdependence of people and their environments; less well understood is the interdependence of women's lives in their three environments—home, community, and workplace. Women's multiple roles spill over from home to community to workplace, so that these environments are in practice inseparable in women's lives. Even when women work outside the home for wages, they still do most of the work of maintaining a home and caring for the family; and almost everywhere women's social skills create and sustain communities, turning women's double day into a triple day. Together these three sets of activities translate into exhaustion, stress, and cumulatively, poor health. This chapter seeks to spell out how sexism, racism, homophobia, and class prejudice mold those environments. Conversely, women's movements shape their environments by mobilizing women to resist and fight back. Women are organizing for change in each of their environments, sometimes in small, everyday protests and sometimes as part of large international movements.

Women's combined experiences of sexism, racism, homophobia, and class prejudice accumulate over a lifetime. Their simultaneous responsibilities in all three environments increase women's workloads and the time they must allot to fulfill their commitments. Every study shows that women work more hours than men each day. When poverty increases women's already heavy work burdens, it also raises their risk of ill health. Infectious diseases (for the most part environmental and still the leading causes of death in the global South) circulate through all of women's activities. The AIDS epidemic, analyzed in the concluding section of this chapter, graphically illustrates this point.

The Home Environment

Sexism dictates the gender dynamics of women's lives at home, including who does the housekeeping, nursing (of the young and old), and childrearing—undervalued, unacknowledged work for which women are not paid when they do it in their own homes. Yet employers compensate men on the assumption that the women in their lives will do this work for them and that men will not have to purchase these services in the marketplace. Sexism also accounts for women's assignment to maintain social relations in the family (and in the community), work that men almost always trivialize as gossip.

A common element of women's lives in every part of the world is the responsibility they bear for running the household and caring for all its members in sickness and health. This household labor is never paid and never ending. The amount of drudgery it entails, in the absence of labor-saving devices, increases as women's caste or class position nears the bottom of the hierarchy, as their home is in a more rural or remote location, and as the level of their community's development sinks. A marginal farming area in Kenya shows disability levels in women aged 20–60 years approximately double those of men. Disability was greater for men only from 15–19 years and over 60 years (Sims and Butter 2000). Of course, the greatest dangers to women and girls at home are domestic violence and sexual abuse including incest and rape (see chapter 5).

In rural areas of the global South, women's daily, most onerous tasks are the collection of water and firewood. Deforestation by logging companies and pollution of water by commercial farms further exacerbate women's workloads, as they have to walk longer distances for fuel and water. The work is physically arduous, the heavy loads cause hip, leg, and shoulder pain, and repeated trips can result in menstrual disorders, miscarriage, and stillbirth (Paolisso and Leslie 1995). In conflict zones, in relocation and refugee camps, these tasks also expose women to the dangers of physical and sexual assault. Women's responsibility for feeding the family exposes them to burns from cooking fires and to pollution from the use of smoky fuels indoors leading to respiratory problems related to smoke inhalation. Indoor air pollution is but one of many hazards women face in the home environment that the state does not regulate because it does not recognize the home as a workplace. Recent evidence suggests that indoor air pollution may be associated not only with greater cardiovascular morbidity in women, but also with higher risks of tuberculosis and higher levels of blindness; it may also interfere with the absorption of nutrients (Sen, George, and Östlin 2002).

When researchers ask women who describe themselves as housewives or homemakers about their health, they speak about the work, chafing at its compulsory nature and workloads that leave no time for rest. Their health suffers, they note, because their tasks are essential to the family's survival. "As for women's work, it's compulsory—no rest . . . You can't say that I'm tired so I won't do this, or I'll postpone it" (interview with Ghanaian woman quoted in Avotri and Walters 1999, 1128). In Africa, where households may not pool incomes, women are typically responsible for the care of their family and for the economic support of their children. They face a precarious financial situation and engage in multiple economic activities to survive. Many of these jobs are home-based and in the informal sector, blurring the distinction between home and workplace. Textile dyeing, car painting and repair, small metal working, pottery, shoe making, and carpentry are all examples of small industries that impose physical and chemical hazards and that are also often located within or very close to home (Sims and Butter 2000).

Since 1972, the International Wages for Housework Campaign, a network of women in Third World and industrialized countries, has organized to get compensation for the unwaged work that women do, with payments coming from a dismantled military-industrial complex. At the World Conference to Review and Appraise the Achievements of the UN Decade for Women held in Nairobi in 1985, Wages for Housework succeeded in persuading the world's governments to count women's unwaged work in agriculture, food production, reproduction, and household activities in every country's Gross National Product (UN Forward-Looking Strategies 1985). International Black Women for Wages for Housework, an international network of black women, other women of color, immigrant, and migrant women, founded in 1975, organizes in countries of the South and the North against poverty and overwork and for financial compensation for unwaged and low-waged work. It coordinates the International Network of Women of Colour—grassroots activists of Africa, Latin America, Asia/Pacific, and the Caribbean, as well as Native American women—working to ensure that challenges to racism are not separated from or prioritized over challenges to sexism and other forms of discrimination; the goal is to resist divide-and-rule strategies among black people and people of color and to work more effectively with white women and men and men of color who share the groups' aims.

Community Environments

The community environment, whether urban, peri-urban, or rural, is an extension of women's home environment. In rural areas, the community is the center of solidarity and mutuality, or hostility and danger, depending on the cohesion of the community and its tolerance for ethnic, religious, caste, and class diversity. In patriarchal communities and in mixed, mutually hostile, communal environments, unaccompanied women and lesbians may be at high risk of violence. In peri-urban and urban areas, solidarity is likely to vary with the age and stability of the slum (shantytown, *bidonville*, barrio, *favela*). Older communities may develop mutually supportive networks, as in Chile during the Pinochet dictatorship (Scarpaci 1993), or gangs may overrun them, as in Rio de Janeiro (Richardson and Kirsten 2005). Women's position varies in each of these situations, and as the number of women migrating alone from rural to urban areas has increased, women's groups have brought attention to these issues.

Women in the global South play a key role in managing and preserving biodiversity, water, land, and other natural resources, yet governments generally ignore or exploit women's importance to their communities. The links between women and the environment are mostly hidden and need to be made visible. An explicit focus on gender relations could improve the management of resources and create opportunities for greater ecological diversity and food production. SEWA, the Indian women's union for self-employed women, involved women in water management by providing training for pump repair, which yielded additional income-generating activities, constructing roof water tanks and caves for water storage (SEWA 2000). Environmental risks relate to gender-specific work and result in different rates of tropical diseases for women and men. Women are far more likely than men to contract schistosomiasis, a disease caused by a parasite that swims in bodies of water, because they are the family laundresses; when women are responsible for cultivation, they are more vulnerable to malaria and filariasis, two more parasitic diseases; and domestic roles expose women to dengue, Chagas' disease, and leishmaniasis (WHO 1995).[1]

Simultaneously, exposure to the environmental risks of unregulated industrialization is occurring, with virtually no data on industrial sources of persistent toxic substances and a paucity of detailed data on pesticide use (Sims and Butter 2000). In industrial countries, cancer kills one woman out of every three and one man out of every two, and its incidence is increasing at about 1 percent per year (Burdon 2003). About 75 to 80 percent of cancers are due to environmental factors that environmental policies could reduce or even eradicate (heredity alone accounts for only about 10 to 15 percent of an individual's risk of developing cancer). As industrialization changes the environment in many countries of the global South, cancer is becoming a problem where it never was before. In remote villages along China's Shaying River, the number of cancer cases has grown from dozens to hundreds per year since heavy industry came to the river's banks in the 1980s (www.nicholas.duke.edu/think accessed 19 July 2005). One need not work in an industry to be exposed; just sharing an environment with industrial polluters increases one's risk of cancer.

Industrialization in India led to the citing of a Union Carbide fertilizer plant in the center of Bhopal, a city of more than one million. In 1984 the plant erupted killing nearly 3,000 people initially, and an estimated 15,000 to 20,000 from related illnesses since then, and sickening anywhere from 150,000 to 600,000. Twenty years later, women experiencing cancer, infertility, and menstrual irregularities continue to battle for justice. One organization of gas victims that emerged as strong and sustained was the Bhopal Gas-Affected Women Workers' Organization. Not a feminist organization, it is linked to the women's movement, and a number of feminist groups work within it.

Environmental disasters may be a sudden catastrophe like the explosions in Bhopal or Chernobyl and the tsunami of December 2004 or a slow environmental death like the one taking place for over 20 years around the Aral Sea, a region touching five Central Asian countries. Intensive cotton cultivation involving aerial spraying, diversion of feeder rivers for massive irrigation schemes, salt and mineral contamination of the soil, and heavy erosion created a series of environmental, health, and social problems, including significant destruction of livelihoods, massive impoverishment, migration, and the weakening of family and social networks (Sims and Butter 2000).

Indigenous peoples both North and South face high levels of pollution, even as they are highly dependent on ever diminishing natural resources. In Mexico, Yaqui living in a rural area contaminated by toxic pesticides suffer alarming rates of impaired neuromuscular and intellectual development. Accusations of environmental racism in the United States, buttressed by empirical findings that the marginalized suffer disproportionately from environmental risks due to industrial pollution, waste dumps, and occupational exposure, have led indigenous peoples and feminists to join in debates about environmental injustice (Sims and Butter 2000). Women face specific environmental risks due to their biology; for example, women are more susceptible than men to autoimmune conditions, which are connected with environmental estrogens and the fact that hazardous substances accumulate in adipose tissue, which women have more of than men.[2]

International agencies almost always link environmental health issues to economic development. Neoliberal policymakers consider the maintenance of the environment—clear air and clean water (known to economists as common goods or public goods)—an impediment to economic growth; the ability to pollute with impunity allows corporations to externalize the environmental and health costs of doing business. In response, the movement for environmental justice has broadened its attack on polluting corporations and joined forces with protestors demonstrating against economic globalization. In addition to the highly publicized protests in Seattle (1999), Genoa (2001), and Miami (2003), dozens of protest movements have occurred at the national level. Street demonstrations in Argentina, Bolivia, Malaysia, Mexico, Thailand, and South Africa have disrupted meetings of international financial institutions.

Some protestors have directed their anger specifically against polluters that despoil their environment and threaten their survival. On 8 August 2002, Nigerian women from surrounding communities in the Niger Delta occupied Chevron's Escravos oil terminal. The impoverished women, long neglected and forced to bear the burden of pollution-related dwindling harvests and incomes, demanded a clean environment conducive to survival, jobs for their children, hospitals, safe drinking water, and support for livelihood ventures like poultry farming (ERA/FoEN 2002).

Other protestors have targeted destructive environmental practices that threaten their livelihoods. The Chipko movement in the Himalayan foothills of Uttar Pradesh, India, emerged in 1972–1974 when peasants hugged the trees in their communities to prevent loggers from cutting them down. Women were prominent in these actions, and in the 1980s the public knew Chipko as a women's movement (Omvedt 1993). Women understood that green trees are critical to the water cycle, and they focused on the function of water in producing, maintaining, and improving soil structure. Two decades later, Vandana Shiva,[3] the prominent

Indian environmental activist, launched Navdanya through her Research Foundation for Science, Technology, and Ecology. Navdanya responds to corporate monopolies promoting monoculture (the cultivation of single crops over large areas) by facilitating seed conservation and the exchange of traditional seed varieties among local groups and communities (Cerón, Das, and Fort 2004).

Another approach is citizen self-assessment in which women are leaders (Breton 1998). Community health diagnoses are a way to study environmental health effects at the community level that includes collecting information on disease clusters and providing early warning to public authorities. Health professionals can follow up by testing the blood and urine of community members in the most contaminated areas to assess the degree of contamination. Southeast Asian and African environmental NGOs are interested in the use of volunteers to administer questionnaires and register both health complaints and environmental circumstances (Sims and Butter 2000).

North/South collaboration has emerged between local groups: the California-based Filipino-American Coalition for Environmental Solutions (FACES) worked in solidarity with Filipino activists to force the U.S. Department of Defense to conduct environmental assessments at former military bases that have contaminated the environment causing illness and death in Filipinos exposed to toxic wastes (Cerón, Das, and Fort 2004). The Women's Health and Environments Network (WHEN), based in Toronto, is a coalition of Canadian organizations dedicated to increasing awareness and actions that reduce toxic risks to environmental contaminants. Since 1994, WHEN has been educating the media, policymakers, and the general public about environmental health as a key determinant of public health. They focus on primary prevention of environmentally linked health problems such as cancer, asthma, and conditions related to the immune system. WHEN advocates reduction of toxic emissions, a shift to safe production models, biological agriculture, and biological lawn care; it also calls for more efficient, renewable energy sources and affordable public transportation (WGNRR 2001a, 29–30).

The Workplace Environment

The rapid changes occurring in women's economic roles in the global South create additional health risks for women and further differentiate their health needs from those of men and those of their family (Paolisso and Leslie 1995). Women account for 40 percent of the labor force worldwide, evidence of the "feminization" of the labor force. When the trend started in the 1960s, the high rate of women's employment in export-processing industries represented a radical departure for multinational corporations and another stage in the search for cheap labor (Safa 1986). Expansion of market economies brought opportunities for paid work in the formal and informal sectors and perhaps new autonomy for women, but the terms and conditions of employment have been deteriorating. Employers have lowered labor costs and sidestepped social security obligations and labor laws, with serious repercussions for women's health (Molyneux and Razavi 2006).

Women work at construction sites and do heavy farm work, bent under loads of bricks or bundles of fodder while balancing babies tied to their back. (Myths about women being the weaker sex do not apply here.) Work in commercial agriculture exposes women to toxic pesticides in cash crop farming. Pesticide Action Network (PAN) studied eight Asian countries and found that more than 90 percent of the women regularly spray pesticides without adequate protection, often while carrying a baby on their back; many cannot read labels, and tasks like weeding, cleaning equipment and clothing, and disposal of leftovers expose all of them. Long working hours in factories expose women to carcinogenic substances and a fast, intense pace at monotonous, repetitive tasks in stressful, sometimes threatening, situations. In these conditions, eyesight deteriorates on assembly lines in the electronics industry. Women's health risks at work tend to be relatively invisible compared to the more dramatic and more frequently fatal hazards that men face (Messing and de Grosbois 2001), and governments fail to regulate the conditions most frequently hazardous to women.

Sexism controls women's productive waged labor, beginning with educational discrimination that denies girls the same opportunities as boys and limits women's choice of occupation. Once in the workplace, employers discriminate against women in assignments, promotions, and pay. Sexual harassment, violence, and sexist discrimination add to the stress associated with competing roles at home and at work. If women leave the workforce temporarily to bear and raise children, employers penalize them in seniority or they lose their job security. Fewer women than men are unionized or work in unionized workplaces; unionization affects pay scales and grievance procedures. Women of color often work in invisible jobs—as domestics, in the food industry, in the lower echelons of the health industry. The assumptions remain (against all evidence) that women work only until they get married or have a child, and that women work for "pin" money—for the extras over and above the wages that their husbands bring home. The cumulative result is lower lifetime pay, lower pensions, more poverty, and more ill health in old age.

In the past 35 years, activists and trade unionists have pressed governments to redefine the field of occupational safety and health, which now covers the workplace environment, occupational illness and injuries, and women. Under pressure from the occupational health movement, government regulators added occupational hazards and environmental risks to the field of workplace safety, once narrowly defined as injury prevention and for too long the only health concern of plant managers. Countries that adopted legislation to protect working women on the grounds that men's work is dangerous and they should not expose women to such risks, effectively excluded women from better paying jobs[4] and allowed companies to avoid the expense of making the workplace an environment safe for all workers.

Women of color (North and South) are at even more risk in jobs where female workforces predominate: nursing, small parts assembly, office work, and agriculture. Gender inequities in occupational health occur when women work in jobs that are more unhealthy than those men do and when jobs remain unhealthy because mainly women do them. The ergonomics of women's work is different from that of men's, in part because men design the machines and tools that men handle. Most women are smaller and lighter than the average man in their societies, and women's upper body strength is not as great as men's; hence women need differently designed machines and tools of smaller sizes. Governments' failure to observe the ergonomics of women's work in repetitive assembly jobs results in disorders of the skeleton and muscles associated with repetition, overuse, and constrained work postures.

Three levels of control are available to limit the risks of occupational injury and illness: engineering controls, administrative controls, and behavioral controls. Managers can enlist workers in making changes and to introducing new designs to reduce risk of injury. Poor work organization can lead to job stress, which also raises the likelihood of injury. Rotating through a variety of tasks is one way to reduce the degree of hazard (see table 3.1).

Sexism, Racism, and Class Prejudice
in the Workplace

Gender-based occupational segregation is an enduring characteristic of labor markets in all countries, irrespective of the level of economic

Table 3.1 Work related health risks for women at home, in the community, and at work

Health problem	Gender specific/gender related cause
Burns	Women's responsibility for meal preparation on open stoves or fires
Smoke pollution: cough dyspnoea, respiratory abnormalities, detrimental effects on fetal growth	Cooking in poorly ventilated structures using biomass fuel sources
Sore and painful, legs, hips, and shoulders, and fatigue	Carrying heavy loads like water, firewood, and harvests
Prolapsed uterus, miscarriage, stillbirth	Carrying heavy loads like water, firewood, and harvests
Physical and sexual assault	Domestic violence, poor community facilities (latrines, street lighting, policing), lack of safe transport to and from workplaces
Chronic back pain and leg problems	Work in small-farm subsistence agriculture: weeding, transplanting, threshing, postharvest processing
Exposure to toxic pesticides (with effects on fetuses and breastfed infants)	Cash crop production: prolonged exposure through hand labor, weeding, picking, and sorting, in sprayed fields; lack of protective equipment and clothing
Factory hazards to health and safety and exposure to carcinogens, acids, solvents, and gases	Assembly line production: long shifts; fast paced, intensive, monotonous, repetitive work
Byssinosis (brown lung)	Work in clothing industry; exposure to textile lint
Eye problems, loss of eyesight	Electronic assembly line work

Source: Adapted from Paolisso and Leslie 1995.

development, the political system, or the religious, social, or cultural environment (UN 2000b). Women are segregated in certain types of work (sometimes called horizontal segregation) and are congregated at the bottom of work hierarchies in both male and female occupations (vertical segregation); the differences between women and men in the same occupation in terms of grade, pay, authority, and career options are also systematic (Östlin 2002).

Extensive sex stereotyping in the formal economy of Peru derives in part from implicit or explicit sex discrimination. Factors that influence employers to discriminate are the *machista* pattern of patriarchy in the Peruvian upper and middle classes, the gender ideology of foreign entrepreneurs operating in Peru, and technological changes that embody gender assumptions about the place of women in certain manual jobs (Scott 1990). These patterns work against women from traditional peasant areas that do not share the class-based and patriarchal assumptions of the urban bourgeoisie.

In the United States, racism and sexism affect the health of black and Latina women workers by subjecting them to harassment and discrimination that affect their physical and psychological health, control and limit their place in the workforce hierarchy, and block promotions and reduce pay, with long-term effects on pensions, old-age security, and health. Racism and sexism exclude women from some lines of work, often the best paid. Sometimes racism and sexism operate so early in life in the educational system that girls never receive the basic training they need to enter certain occupations.

When these scenarios conspire to limit the advancement of women of color in the upper echelons of the health professions, the result is that all women's health care suffers. When the establishment denies women physicians and nurses positions of responsibility in government and in the academy, these women do not reach posts in which they could influence policy. And when medical schools do not train women who come from disadvantaged communities, those communities suffer; we know that people who come from such communities are more likely to return and serve their community than are elite physicians.

Class prejudice also plays a role in creating hierarchies among women workers. In the United States, where talk about social class is less common than in many other countries, the government uses income or race as a proxy for social class. Income and race shift our focus away from the causes and consequences of poverty to individual characteristics and victim blaming. Great Britain has used social class to organize data on population health and occupational health since the early 1900s. The British government defines social class according to occupational categories as laid out in table 3.2.[5]

In every study undertaken in Great Britain (and the British have documented occupational health according to social class since 1911), there is a positive correlation between health and social class: the higher the class, the better the health. Even when overall health in society improves over time, the gap between social classes does not close. Access to health services is not the issue since the National Health Service covers everyone.

This classification of workers does not allow us to extrapolate the health of women workers in countries that do not keep such tallies, partly because the categories reflect occupational status in British society rather than an objective measure of economic class. In most regions (excepting sub-Saharan Africa and Southern Asia), women work primarily in the service sector. In the British categorization, service work

Table 3.2   Social classes in Great Britain

Social Class I Professionals	Physicians, engineers, architects, scientists, large employers, directors of business (CEOs) (these workers receive annual salaries and benefits)
Social Class II Lower professionals	Teachers, pharmacists, social workers, and managers (these workers receive annual salaries and benefits); authors, owners of small businesses, and farmers (these workers are often self-employed)
Social Class III	a) Nonmanual skilled workers Artisans, white collar workers (office and clerical workers) (their terms of remuneration often depend on unionization) b) Manual skilled workers Supervisors, (for example, in factories), transport workers (their terms of remuneration often depend on unionization)
Social Class IV	Partly skilled workers, semi-skilled factory workers, agricultural laborers, service workers★
Social Class V	Unskilled workers: laborers, domestic servants, casual workers (workers in this category receive minimum wages, no benefits, no job security)

★ Note how far down the scale service workers are—service work is the largest growing occupational field in many countries.

falls into social class IV, but the UN (2000) includes a broader range of activity in the service category than does Great Britain; for example, the UN includes as services public administration, social security, defense, education, health, and social work, which correspond to social class II. Similarly, in sub-Saharan Africa and Southern Asia, the agricultural sector has the highest proportion of women (65 percent); but the UN does not tell us whether these jobs are comparable to "farmer" (social class II) or "agricultural laborer" (social class IV).

Maquila and Free Trade Zone Workers

The following sections highlight briefly the problems of special categories of women workers: women in maquiladoras and free trade zones, immigrant workers, domestic workers, women who are trafficked, women in sex work, and pregnant workers. Women isolated in domestic work and in sex work on the streets face special dangers, with little police protection and few effective legal protections despite many recorded violations of labor laws. Women are organizing to combat harmful situations in almost every country in which they occur.

Maquiladoras are foreign-owned assembly plants in Mexico (the term now extends to Central America). Companies import machinery and materials duty free and export finished products around the world. The lax enforcement of environmental laws allows many plants to pollute with impunity, creating hazardous air and water conditions for nearby communities. One of the worst cases, an abandoned battery recycling plant near Tijuana, Mexico, Metales y Derivados, owned by the San Diego-based New Frontier Trading Corporation, illegally stored 7,000 tons of toxic waste in the soil surrounding the plant. The Border Region Workers' Support Committee and the Citizen's Committee for the Restoration of Cañon del Padre documented a growing number of children born with anencephaly (the absence of a major portion of the brain, skull, and scalp, anencephaly is an increasingly frequent birth defect in industrial communities all along the border). Together with the San Diego-based Environmental Health Coalition (EHC), the Citizen's Committee in Tijuana filed a complaint with the administration of the North American Free Trade Agreement (NAFTA). "Nothing changed on the ground," grumbled EHC policy advocate Connie Garcia; "NAFTA provides for no cleanup plan or enforcement mechanism, and the community continues to be poisoned" (quoted in Bacon 2005).

About 60 percent of maquiladora workers are women. Employers make extensive use of racial and sexual stereotypes in both the recruitment of workers and control of the workforce. Employers humiliate male workers by symbolically turning them into women, for example by making them work in the women's section. The underlying message is that employers treat women poorly and with disrespect and that they will treat any man who steps out of line as a woman (HRW 1996; Nathan 1999; Salzinger 2001). Women's groups like La Mujer Obrera (an association of border workers), Ocho de Marzo Women's Rights in Juarez, Mexico, and CODEFAM Marianela Garcia Villa in El Salvador are struggling against unfair labor practices and human rights violations.

Free trade zones (FTZ) are an integral part of several economies in the global South. Working conditions are often dangerous and benefits nonexistent. Many of the workers come from rural areas and are unaware of their labor rights. Under these circumstances, some feminists contend, work contributes to women's oppression rather than their independence. Sri Lanka FTZs employ over 100,000 workers; 75 percent of them are single women between 20 and 29 years old. Though FTZ employers prefer women as workers, their image in society is poor and marriage ads in major Sri Lankan newspapers often state "no factory girls" (https://www.cleanclothes.org/urgent/01-09-23.htm accessed 5 January 2007). Ten to twelve workers share a cramped room 10ft x 12ft, which frequently lacks electricity and fresh water; they cook inside the room although ventilation and sanitation systems are usually inadequate. Sri Lanka does not apply its labor laws in FTZs, where the government does not allow trade unions and bars the International Labor Organization from monitoring the situation; even the National Labour Commission needs permission to enter the zones. The DABINDU (Drops of Sweat) Collective (1999/2000) fights for the rights of workers in Katunayaka and Biyagama; they report on working and living conditions, the harsh punishments meted out for mistakes, harassment in the plants, and sexual violence on the roads between the zones and the boarding houses where the workers live. Together with the Women's Centre, the Joint Committee of FTZ Workers, *Kalape Api* (We of the Zone), the Legal Advice Centre, and *Kamkaru Sevana* (Shelter for Women), DABINDU Collective is fighting for workers' rights and for welfare services, such as a hospital and a cooperative for FTZ workers.

A frequent problem that women workers in both maquiladoras and FTZs encounter is that factory owners and managers resist the women's demands for improvements in working and living conditions. Owners threaten to fire the women if they try to unionize, or they declare bankruptcy, shut the plant down, and move on to another country. Human rights organizations try to defend workers in these situations, but companies, knowing that laborers enjoy few protections, rarely compensate the workers they ditch.

Immigrant Workers

The low status of immigrants combined with women's low status leads to special vulnerability to sexual and racial harassment and caste or class prejudice. The work environment is often hostile to immigrant women. Immigrants work in the lowest paid, most dangerous, dirty jobs. Their youth and lack of working experience in mechanized farm work or in factories exposes immigrants to unfamiliar dangers and makes them more prone to accidents and injuries. Some are poorly educated, with no working knowledge of foreign languages. Language barriers, lack of translation of safety manuals, and an inability to understand verbal warnings shouted in a foreign language all increase risk. Employers generally exploit immigrant workers who have few rights, less bargaining power, and no union protection. Forms of exploitation include not paying for work or not paying fully; speed ups, which increase the danger of injury especially in mechanized repetitive work; strain injuries like carpal tunnel syndrome and knife wounds in meat packing plants; and racial and sexual harassment (Broadway 1994; Stull 1994). Employers routinely deny benefits, do not pay sick leave, and do not organize access to specialized clinics that can deal knowledgeably with the common problems of their occupation. Some are fly-by-night companies that do not observe labor regulations, including occupational health standards and safety regulations. Few countries have enough inspectors to cover all workplaces.

Immigrants often live far from their workplaces, and the commute (rarely in a private car they own) lengthens the workday; some pay their labor contractors to drive them in vans that no inspector has tested, and the rate of injuries in crashes is high. Some work more than one job. The cumulative result is extreme fatigue, which can increase the risk of work accidents. Affordable housing is a headache everywhere, and employers do not pay immigrants enough to cover decent housing and nourishing food. Overcrowding and consumption of "empty calories" may contribute to poor general states of health or may aggravate preexisting conditions like tuberculosis. Immigrants generally work in the secondary sector for employers (or jobbers to whom the work is subcontracted) whose profit margins are small and who, for that reason, cannot afford to provide amenities in the workplace like water fountains and toilets.

Undocumented workers face especially difficult situations because they fear deportation if they complain about dangerous assignments. Employers use workers' lack of documents to exploit them. In general, immigrant workers live in greater economic insecurity than the native born and suffer more stress as a result; combined with the social stress of separation from extended family and friends and the political consequences of nonrepresentation, these insecurities can spell chronic disease. Studies show a high correlation between heavy responsibility, little autonomy or authority, and heart disease. A poignant account of the struggles of Vietnamese refugee women working in a beef packing plant in the United States details the economic and health insecurity of lives divided between work demands and family responsibilities; these women subsidize industry costs by adapting to company time and labor controls (Benson 1994).

Pregnancy presents special problems for immigrant women who may have no access to prenatal care or assistance in delivery. Employers rarely grant them rest periods or lighter work to compensate for pregnancy; mothers may be unable to breastfeed or arrange care for other children. Public health outreach to immigrants is not very effective, particularly when it comes to tackling harmful cultural practices; agencies tend to leave the task to community groups. Health workers often neglect communities of recent immigrants because of the variety of languages spoken, and women are less likely to learn the host language than are men.

Despite all these obstacles, immigrant workers have historically been in the forefront of unionization. Many immigrant groups organized in the twentieth century in the United States: European Americans in the American Federation of Labor, Chinese in the Chinese Seamen's Union (1911) and the Chinese Hand Laundry Alliance (1930s), and Mexicans in *mutualistas*; Emma Tenayuca played a leading role in organizing Mexican Americans in San Antonio during the Depression (Louie 2001).

Domestic Workers

Migrant workers and immigrants do domestic work in many countries richer than those they come from. Women and girls from rural areas working as domestics in their own countries find themselves in distant cities, sometimes in extended family systems that treat them as servants rather than as kin. Sexual and physical abuse is rampant in both national and international migratory contexts (HRW 2006).

Trinidadian domestic workers, the majority of whom are single parents, earn half of the legal minimum wage; their employers escape state regulations and employment policies. To give women a forum in which to make their grievance known, the National Union of Domestic Employees, from the mid-1970s, struggled to have the nation's Industrial Relations Act recognize domestic workers (Karides 2002).

In Nigeria, in the past, some parents encouraged their children to live with distant family members in a system based on mutual benefit that excluded cash transfers. The system has changed, become monetized, and the family connection loosened, leading to more abuse, especially of girls. The Hope Project, based in Lagos, works with adolescent girls to educate them about reproductive health and with authorities to develop regulations for domestic employment; the project uses radio broadcasts to disseminate information and gives the girls transistor radios so that they can listen to the programs (Akinrimisi 2003).

After the first Gulf War in 1991, over 2,000 Asians from Sri Lanka, Bangladesh, India, and the Philippines working as maids in Kuwait fled from employers who assaulted them physically and sexually, held them in debt bondage, deprived them of their passports, confined them illegally, and violated their contracts (Women's Rights Project and Middle East Watch 1992). Only one case of abuse was successfully prosecuted, that of Sonia Panama, a 23-year old Filipina working as a maid who died in hospital of severe abuse that included beatings, rape, cigarette burns covering her body, a virtually severed ear, and bite marks on her stomach. The court sentenced her employers, a Kuwaiti husband and Lebanese wife, to seven years in prison for causing her death through ill treatment (HRW 1993a, 363–364).

Sex Work and Trafficking

Not all trafficking is for sex work and not all smuggling of people is trafficking. Some migrant workers or would-be immigrants arrange for their own smuggling; others are trafficked against their will. In both cases, women may end up in near-slave conditions of debt bondage, held against their will with little means of escape. And the threat of AIDS is now an occupational hazard, affecting sex workers everywhere.

Sex work and the trafficking of women to work in the sex industry encompass a wide and varied range of activity. At one end is the willing agreement of women to work as prostitutes whom intermediaries or employers may cheat after they begin work, and the duping of women anxious to migrate to wealthier countries or escape a dead-end situation at home. At the other end is the kidnapping of young girls to work in brothels and the purchase of daughters from naive or knowing parents. Analysis of the problems of sex work and the trafficking of women and girls is complex; among contributing factors are the discrimination that women endure, their lack of opportunity, the poverty in which so many live out their lives, the unceasing demand for sexual services, and the large sums that purveyors of sex reap from the sale of women's bodies. The new social order of globalization manipulates women economically, often drawing them into dangerous situations and depriving them of safe and secure means of migration, decent employment at home or abroad, and education (Limanowska 2001).

Because sex work and trafficking arouse outrage, many groups have mounted campaigns against it. Some campaigns, like the Thai government's widely publicized crackdown on child prostitution, are official, mounted at the national level; some receive international cooperation. Others are nongovernmental efforts: Thai Friends of Women began as a women's information center in 1984 to counsel women who were seeking employment overseas on the problems they might encounter, especially in the sex industry abroad (Tantiwiramanond and Pandey 1991). For the past dozen years, sex work traffickers have targeted women of the former Soviet Union and the countries of Eastern and Central Europe; most of them trick women into taking a job that turns out to be prostitution and they hold the women against their will (HRW 2004). A network of traffickers moves the women across borders and ethnic communities, part of a web that spreads across the Balkans and into Western Europe (Gall 2001; see also http://www.stopvaw.org/Trafficking_in_Women.html accessed 21 March 2007).

The Women's Rights Project of Human Rights Watch and Asia Watch documented the trafficking of 20,000 to 30,000 Burmese women and girls to Thailand in the early 1990s. Held in bondage for debts incurred in their recruitment, transportation, and living expenses, girls as young as 11 and 12 were forced into brothels to have sex with 10 to 15 men a day (HRW 1993b). Human Rights Watch implicated corrupt Thai police as drivers, procurers, and protection racketeers who were indifferent to the deplorable conditions of the Burmese and failed to enforce the law. When police did raid the brothels, they arrested the women and girls and held them in overcrowded detention centers where they sometimes raped and physically abused them before deporting them to Burma. The Thai police rarely arrested brothel owners, pimps, and traffickers and prosecuted them even less often. HIV infected an estimated 50 to 70 percent of the Burmese women in Thailand, and the Thai government knew that the Burmese persecute people with AIDS, that deportation carried a death sentence.

In India today, after years of effort, the sex workers of Sonagachi (Calcutta) are able to negotiate safer sex relationships with clients and better treatment from society, including the police (Bala Nath 2000). In 1992 the STD/HIV Intervention Project (SHIP) set up a sexually transmitted disease clinic for sex workers to promote disease control and condom distribution. They soon broadened their focus to address structural issues of gender, class, and sexuality. The sex workers themselves decide the program's strategies. Of managerial positions, 25 percent are reserved for sex workers who hold many key positions and act as peer educators, clinic assistants, and clinic attendants in the project's STD clinics.

SHIP conducted a survey with the sex workers using participatory methodology. The survey confirmed that extreme economic poverty and social deprivation were the main reasons women became involved in the sex trade. Once sex workers saw the results of the survey and the survey statistics, they could see their vulnerability in the context of structural problems, and those who previously had negative self-images began to change their perspective. The peer educators went from house to house in red-light districts carrying information on STD/HIV prevention, how to access medical care, and ways to question power structures that promote violence (Bala Nath 2000). They conducted a survey with *babus* (long-term regular clients); only half had heard of AIDS and three-fourths had never used a condom. The sex workers formed alliances with their clients to promote safer sexual practices and to eliminate sexual violence in the area. Together with the All India Institute of Health and Hygiene they trained police from the Calcutta Police Department. SHIP also responds to the needs of the sex workers as they arise, providing informal education, vocational training programs for security in old age, and a credit and savings scheme to help sex workers become self-employed (Bala Nath 2000). Sex workers set up the Komal Gandhar theatre group, through which they were able to communicate publicly methods of negotiating safer sex with clients, pimps, the police, and brothel owners in a nonthreatening environment. In 1995, they formed a union for sex workers: the Durbar Mahila Samanvaya Committee (DMSC) promotes and enforces their rights (Bala Nath 2000). The state government formally recognizes the regulatory board that DMSC members set up with a couple of state departments to ensure that everyone involved in the red-light areas of West Bengal adheres to the mutually agreed code of conduct. Negotiating with the government and with groups of pimps and brothel owners, the sex workers are directly challenging oppressive structures and patriarchal domination.

As in India, Cambodian sex workers have formed a union. The Cambodian Prostitutes Union recommends recognition of sex work as a legitimate occupation, benefiting from protective legislation that will eliminate exploitation and that will give sex workers full profit from their work. They recommend decriminalization of sex work so that sex workers will have the power to protect themselves. They want an end to police harassment, abuse, and violence (WGNRR 2000a). Other NGOs come close to the principle of unionization in their work with prostitutes; for instance, the Thai NGO EMPOWER works to protect bar girls' rights and to give them the skills they need to take control of their lives (Tantiwiramanond and Pandey 1991).

In Bangladesh, the Prime Minister allocated $400,000 to evict sex workers from Tanbazar and Nimtoli, large brothels located 25 kilometers south of Dhaka, the capital. Twenty-three organizations took up the cause of the 1,600 women working in Tanbazar, including the Bangladesh Women's Health Coalition, the Bangladesh Association of Women for Self-Empowerment, Ulka (association of evicted sex workers of Kandupatti brothel), Durjoy (association of floating sex workers of Dhaka), and Mukti (sex workers from a brothel in Tangail); they demanded that the government not force the sex workers of Tanbazar and Nimtoli out of their homes and professions (WGNNR 1999/2000).

Labor Laws: Maternity Protection, Fetal "Rights"

The history of special protection for women workers is as old as the first public health responses to the Industrial Revolution. The tension between protection (recognition of women's special needs in pregnancy and lactation) and discrimination (depriving women of the better-paid jobs offered to men and failure to make the workplace safe for all) is a theme common to all women's labor struggles.

In South Korea, women campaigned successfully for the reform of laws regulating the work of women (Wang 2002).[6] Among the groups waging the campaign to achieve socialization of maternity protection costs are the Korean Women Workers Associations United (KWWAU), which submitted petitions, held open public discussions and rallies, and released hundreds of statements. In the past, employers were largely responsible for maternity costs; they fired women workers when they married, became pregnant, and bore children or they forcibly reassigned them to areas distant from their families in an effort to discourage them from continuing to work. Korean law limited maternity leave to 60 days (the International Labor Organization recommends 14 weeks). Beyond maternity leave, KWWAU moved to make the workplace safer for women of childbearing age and lobbied for protections in the handling of dangerous chemicals. The women also won a stronger Equal Employment Act, which now extends to workplaces with fewer than five workers, has stronger measures against discriminatory employers, and better protects women against sexual harassment. The new act also expands paid leave for the purpose of childcare for all workers (not just mothers) and makes reinstatement in previous positions mandatory.

Issues of fetal "rights" in industrial settings in the United States followed the Supreme Court ruling to legalize abortion in 1973. Many companies, concerned about liability from workers' lawsuits, barred all women of childbearing age from jobs exposing them to toxins that might harm a fetus; this practice jeopardized women's access to some 15 to 20 million industrial, relatively high-paying, blue-collar jobs. The formula companies used posed a false conflict between the right of a fetus to health and a woman's right to employment opportunity. Their real project was to pit the company's drive for profit against a woman's economic right to a job that does not harm her health. The companies barred women of childbearing age based on their potential fertility, not actual pregnancy. American Cyanamid implemented a fetal protection policy in 1979 at its plant in Willow Island, West Virginia. Four young women, wanting to work in the lead battery section for higher pay, had their doctors perform hysterectomies so they could prove to the company that they were sterile. OCAW (the Oil, Chemical and Atomic Workers International Union), representing workers at the plant, challenged the policy under the Occupational Safety and Health Act (OSHA) of 1970. Although the Secretary of Labor held with OCAW that the fetal protection policy violated the general duty clause of OSHA, which enjoins employers to furnish employment and a place of employment free from recognized hazards that can cause death or serious physical harm, the Occupational Safety and Health Review Commission overturned the ruling and found that American Cyanamid's policy did not constitute the kind of hazard Congress had in mind when it passed OSHA (Roth 2000).

Following the comparable worth campaign for equal pay for equal work and trade union activism on occupational safety and health, the Supreme Court invalidated so-called fetal protection policies in 1991. In *United Auto Workers* v. *Johnson Controls*, the Supreme Court ruled for a group of workers and their union that challenged a company policy keeping all women up to age 70 out of jobs working with lead (as well as jobs from which women could be promoted to one involving lead) unless they could provide medical proof that they could not become pregnant (Roth 2000). For 20 years society had censured women for not protecting their fetuses and allowed companies to delay cleaning up the workplace or providing alternative work for women (and men) planning to have children. Such victim-blaming attitudes also protect the medical profession and drug companies from liability for the harm they do. Blaming women for damage to the fetus privatizes responsibility for the next generation, placing the onus on women and letting society off the hook for failing to provide better medical care, drug treatment for addicts, and safer workplaces. The focus on the fetus reduces women to incubators and personifies the fetus at the woman's expense.

AIDS, a Syndrome that Bridges Home, Community, and Workplace Environments

Globally AIDS, the autoimmune deficiency syndrome, affects more women than men, although the U.S. Centers for Disease Control and Prevention (CDC) initially defined AIDS as a gay male disease. In the early years of the international epidemic, CDC and the World Health Organization (WHO) paid little attention to women's experiences. Yet they now say that the dominant risk factor for contracting HIV, the virus that causes AIDS, is heterosexual sex, and UNAIDS (2006), which is the joint United Nations program on HIV/AIDS, estimates that almost 50 per cent of those living with HIV are now women (the figure is closer to 60 percent in sub-Saharan Africa). HIV and AIDS now affect women disproportionately as patients and in their social roles as mothers and caregivers. The epidemic is entrenching unequal gender relations and other inequalities implicated as causes.

AIDS affects women disproportionately because most women have little knowledge of how HIV is transmitted before they receive the diagnosis. In both Thailand and Zimbabwe, the little that women did know was based on persistent, contradictory, but common myths about AIDS: that it is a disease of men; that heterosexual transmission of AIDS is rare; that condoms are foolproof protection; that women's promiscuity causes AIDS; and that women are vectors of HIV. Scientists debate the last two of these notions as the evidence shows male to female transmission is twice as likely as female to male transmission. Another reason AIDS affects women disproportionately is that forces such as poverty and gender inequality are the strongest enhancers of risk for exposure to HIV. Although many biomedical and social scientists would agree with this analysis, both groups tend to neglect systemic economic, social, and political factors in their research, concentrating instead on the biological and behavioral aspects of the syndrome.

AIDS is a syndrome that bridges women's three environments—home, community, and workplace. AIDS affects women at home as wives of men who secretly have sex with infected men or women or who inject drugs intravenously, exposing them to HIV. Wives who are not privy to this information cannot without violating social taboos question their husbands, let alone act to protect themselves by demanding the use of condoms. The community enters the picture in several ways: by enforcing social taboos (for example a husband who beats a wife who refuses sex will find support in the community for exercising his marital rights); by becoming the site of HIV transmission because it is impoverished, in a conflict zone, situated on a long-distance trucking route where overnight stops and prostitution are common, or because it is a setting of illegal drug production or export, often associated with drug use. Married men in these communities are at high risk of contracting HIV and transmitting it to their wives at home; and single and married women trying to earn a bit of cash and caught up in these rings are at risk of contracting HIV. AIDS bridges home, community, and workplace when the worksite is a mine or plantation with housing for single migrants who have homosexual relations with other workers or heterosexual relations with women in the surrounding community and then bring the infection home to their wives. Work acts as a bridge when it is service in the armed forces and men who live in barracks seek casual sex. When the workplace is a clinical facility treating people with AIDS but has too few gloves, masks, syringes, needles, and autoclaves to ensure protection against infection, workers may contract HIV. In any of these workplaces, workers may transmit HIV to the communities they live in and to their partners at home.

AIDS at Home

Domestic violence is the clearest danger for women at home; it also increases women's risk of contracting AIDS. A South African study found that women with violent or controlling male partners are at increased risk of HIV infection, probably because abusive men are more likely to have HIV and impose risky sexual practices on their partners (Dunkle et al. 2004). (Interestingly, they also found that child sexual assault, forced first intercourse, and adult sexual assault by nonpartners were not associated with HIV serostatus.)

Infidelity is a taboo subject, yet "transactional" sexual relationships that are long-term but not necessarily exclusive are all too common in many impoverished communities (Manjate, Chapman, and Cliff 2000). The International Center for Research on Women studied women from 10 countries, noting that many expressed concern about the infidelities of their partners but were resigned to their lack of control over the situation; "Women from India, Jamaica, Papua New Guinea, Zimbabwe and Brazil report that raising the issue of their partners' infidelity can jeopardise their physical safety and family stability" (Gupta and Weiss 1993, 405). In Southern Africa, the migrant labor and apartheid systems destabilized family life and probably caused the pattern of concurrent sexual relationships that overlap for months or even years. Women in these relationships expect material support from their partner and are willing to tolerate abuse, including infidelity, for the financial aid (Epstein 2004).

AIDS complicates the home life of women who contract the disease. In many countries, men with AIDS receive treatment before women with AIDS do, and families may hesitate to send women to clinics for fear of disrupting the household duties and care that women provide, including tending to other family members with AIDS. Infected women who become pregnant can transmit HIV during gestation and birth and through breast milk, though the rate of maternal-fetal transmission is low—between 15 and 30 percent. HIV positive women report judgmental and hostile attitudes from service providers, feel that they lose control over their reproductive choices, and complain that health workers test them without asking their consent or refuse to provide services (Manchester and Mthembu 2002). Women living with HIV who request termination of pregnancy report that health workers force them to consent to sterilization (Mthembu 1998). Positively Women (www.positivelywomen.org.uk), a London-based charity that offers peer support to women living with HIV, reported that several women mentioned the negative attitude of doctors toward them becoming pregnant, saying that they would die of AIDS and so would the baby. In African countries, where motherhood establishes a woman's social standing, medical advice not to conceive or breastfeed can have dramatic consequences. Where breastfeeding is a cultural norm, a decision not to breastfeed can lead to disclosure of a woman's HIV status. In overcrowded and overpopulated conditions, a poor woman has less privacy and her neighbors may notice her failure to breastfeed, drawing the conclusion that she is HIV positive.

Prejudices about women's sexuality hinder physicians from diagnosing AIDS in the elderly because they consider them a low-risk group (Ogu and Wolfe 1994). In the United States and Western Europe, 10 percent of AIDS cases occur among people over the age of 50 (UNAIDS 2002). During a recent five-year period, the number of new cases in the over-50 age group increased by 40 percent, with older women having a higher incidence than older men, yet women 15 to 44 years old are the focus of most studies. Physiological changes that occur during menopause, including thinning of the vaginal walls and reduced lubrication, increase older women's vulnerability to HIV. Failure to diagnose the disease in this age group affects the women who suffer from it; the neglect also affects future research done on older women, especially questions of treatment in the elderly who often have more than one concurrent health problem requiring drugs.

AIDS affects women at home in other ways, even those who are not infected. African families may evict the wives and children of their son or brother who died of AIDS, taking over his land, house, and other property, leaving widows homeless and destitute. Customary and sometimes statutory inheritance laws permit this, although in communities that practice levirate marriage, brothers should assume responsibility for widows and their orphaned children. Deepening poverty, in the wake of conflict and economic adjustment programs, has deprived many African men of the ability to fulfill their obligations. Women's groups have had some success working with village leaders and training mediators in property disputes; they have founded groups of village women who counsel new widows on ways to protect their homes and guard their belongings while mourning (*New York Times* editorial 16 June 2004). One group in Kenya, the Obwanda Distress Relief Club, is fighting the practice of levirate marriage on the grounds that uninfected women may be forced to marry infected brothers-in-law and fall ill (Muthengi 2003).

AIDS in the Community

Denial, blame, stigmatization, prejudice, and discrimination are present in every country. Today, AIDS is stigmatizing in the way epidemic diseases were in the past: leprosy since biblical times, tuberculosis in the nineteenth century, cancer in the twentieth. Analyses of stigma seldom focus on how society stigmatizes men and women differently or how women experience such stigma. We know from anecdotal accounts that women and girls who disclose their HIV status risk physical and emotional abuse from communities as well as from partners and family members. In December 1998, members of her community beat to death a young South African woman, Gugu Dlamini, after she disclosed her HIV status; they said she had disgraced the community (Vetten and Bhana 2001).

AIDS carries the additional stigma of racism. Racial prejudice is found in unsubstantiated speculation about where AIDS originated (supposedly in Africa, long before any research could verify that); in how HIV is spread (researchers like Caldwell, Quigley, and Quigley [1989] accused blacks of being sexually promiscuous and said that African sexuality is so different from Euro-Asian norms that it is tantamount to an alternative civilization); in clinical practice and clinical drug trials (researchers gave all U.S. women AZT in drug trials to interrupt maternal transmission, but they gave placebos to some pregnant African women [HRG 1997]); in the very definition of a case of AIDS (in Africa no positive HIV test is needed; diagnosis is based on symptoms [fever, persistent cough, weight loss, and diarrhea] that are common to many diseases); and in the way agencies report the numbers, combining infection (HIV) and disease (AIDS), which inflates the figures. AfricaAction, a Washington-based NGO that is leading a campaign for aid to control AIDS in Africa, calls the neglected epidemic in Africa emblematic of global racism, because the white peoples of the North are neglecting nonwhite people with AIDS in the South.

The relation between racism in the community and AIDS in the home environment is complex. Conservative religious communities do not construct a sound bridge between home and community when they condemn homosexuality or forbid the use of condoms. Their focus on controlling sexuality and sexual behavior deflects attention from institutional and structural forces that impoverish communities and are the ultimate causes of the epidemic. How AIDS plays out in communities is traceable to historical legacies of the slave trade, segregation, and economies of inequality, as well as competitive business practices that deny a living wage to workers. Structural forces constrain individual agency, limiting the choices that a person has; they also determine social status and deny people of low status access to the fruits of science and social progress. Nearly all explanations of AIDS arbitrarily constrict the social field of study, generating the illusion of equally shared risk. Statements about a certain community's denial of risk implicate cultural and psychological factors said to explain AIDS, but they are not etiological descriptions of sources of increased risk. Similar statements pointing to poverty are equally unrevealing since no one willfully lives poor. Nor is poverty a fixed condition or a vicious cycle; it is a product of policies, and governments can change policies. If a government provides jobs when industry will not or cannot, or an income to those out of work, or if it provides free health and education services and free housing, poor people can still live decently, in dignity. Policies that privatize health services, make education unaffordable, and eliminate public housing reinforce the structural forces that create poverty, institutionalize racism and sexism, and deny jobs and income to some groups of people. Such policies destroyed a community in the South Bronx of New York City, paving the way for an AIDS epidemic.

In the 1970s, New York City experienced a severe financial crisis. Unemployment was high, tax revenues were low, businesses (especially manufacturing) were moving out of the city, and New York was near defaulting on its loans. The city adopted a series of policies known in the global South as structural adjustment programs. An austerity budget was a major feature, including cutbacks in education, housing, health services, policing, and firefighting. The municipal government did not distribute these cutbacks equitably across social classes and races in geographically segregated New York City. The cuts fell most heavily on poor residents of color in areas like the South Bronx. Private bank policies reinforced public cutbacks, redlining these districts and refusing to give loans for mortgages, construction, and businesses in them (Wallace and Wallace 1998).

The unemployed failed to pay rent, which meant that the landlords could not pay their mortgages. Banks would not give new loans for new mortgages or repairs in redlined districts. Some landlords simply abandoned their buildings; for others, collecting insurance was a last resort, and they hired arsonists to torch their buildings. But with firehouses closed, the fires burned out of control, and neither the fire department nor the police department (both enduring cutbacks) could pursue or prosecute arsonists. Communities broke apart, not just because fires made people homeless but also because displacement disrupted human networks that constitute neighborhoods. Communities that had watched over local heroin addicts, criminals, and prostitutes (and every neighborhood knew who their problem residents were) were now powerless to control the drug dealers who set up in the burnt-out shells of tenements.

Into this scene came crack cocaine, some say as a result of CIA dealings in Central America (Webb 1996). The crack epidemic hit in ways the heroin epidemic had not: crack was cheaper, more immediately addictive, more women used it, and addicted women started trading sex for drugs. Truck drivers from across the country using the New Jersey turnpike drove across the George Washington Bridge from the Vince Lombardi rest stop (a major center for prostitution) when they heard that crack and women were available cheap in the South Bronx. In the absence of police and neighborhood surveillance, the crack industry flourished, creating jobs for unemployed youth.

Hard on the heels of crack came HIV, into a population already below the poverty line, already overcrowded because families had doubled up to accommodate members made homeless by fires, already discouraged by the relentless rejection of racists and racist institutions.

The Wallace and Wallace (1998) investigation uncovers the devastating conditions that created the AIDS epidemic in the South Bronx and shows that they were not inherent in black people or in black culture but rooted in policies that deprive poor communities of color the public resources necessary for them to function on even the most basic level. Countless communities in Africa, Asia, and Latin America exhibit the same process of disintegration, with different details: substitute structural adjustment programs for the budget cutbacks of New York City, substitute war and armed conflict for arson and fires burning out of control in the South Bronx, substitute soldiers for long-haul truckers and arms dealers for drug kingpins, and substitute sex traffickers who buy or kidnap young girls for addicts and prostitutes (Turshen 1995).

Community responses to the AIDS epidemic have been powerful. The need to change the stigma associated with HIV and AIDS is a major objective of AIDS activists. Another is to accelerate research and treatment. ACTUP (AIDS Coalition to Unleash Power), a largely gay white male organization with a woman's caucus, is one response—a powerful, vocal, effective, and creative element in the international grassroots movement against AIDS. Another is the AIDS Action Coalition that has been relentless in its criticism of the institutions of science and medicine and has not hesitated to intervene from within and without. The interventions of movement activists, beginning at the 1989 International AIDS Conference in Montreal when 300 ACTUP protestors rushed past security brandishing "Silence = Death" placards, significantly changed relationships between mainstream experts and social movements, as well as the practices by which experts manufacture scientific knowledge in society (Epstein 1991). The involvement extends beyond the critique of authority or public policy and into the realm of scientific method and even epistemology. Movement activists maintain that grassroots agents can act on an equal footing with the credentialed experts, can participate in advancing knowledge about AIDS, and, as lay spokespersons, can attain a level of qualification that permits them to speak authoritatively about scientific theories, facts, and methods.

Gender AIDS Forum (GAF) is a Durban-based South African NGO committed to enabling a deeper consciousness in women and men about the links between gender and AIDS. An activist organization committed to transforming an unequal society, GAF places women at the center and believes that "another world is possible" where we are all equal regardless of race, sexual orientation, ethnicity, geographical location, (dis)ability, and gender (http://www.gaf.org.za/ accessed 5 January 2007). The Treatment Action Campaign (TAC) of South Africa, launched in 1998, combats the view that AIDS is a death sentence with education and with demands for universal access to antiretroviral treatment. TAC believes that even poor countries like South Africa can distribute drugs to prolong the life of people with AIDS and reduce the risk of mothers with HIV transferring the virus to their newborn babies. TAC is critical of the pharmaceutical industry for overpricing drugs, for excessive profiteering, and for draconian patent laws.

Other African groups campaigning for those infected and affected by AIDS are TASO, BONELA, and Musasa. Dr. Noerine Kaleeba founded TASO (The AIDS Support Organization) in 1987 with 15 other colleagues, most of whom have since died of AIDS. TASO was based on people unified by the common experiences they faced when encountering AIDS at a time of high stigma, ignorance, and discrimination. Today, TASO is the largest indigenous NGO providing AIDS services in Uganda and the region; it has registered 83,000 people with AIDS, and 22,000 directly receive care and support (http://www.tasouganda.org/ accessed 7 January 2007). BONELA is the Botswana Network on Ethics, Law and AIDS; their mission is to combat stigma by integrating ethical, legal, and human rights dimensions into the national response to the epidemic (Tabengwa 2003). Musasa is a women's rights organization in Zimbabwe that has challenged the discriminatory rules and systems over which authorities have jurisdiction. Musasa has worked with the police and judiciary to develop more sensitive ways of responding to AIDS, as well as to survivors of domestic violence and rape (Butcher and Welbourn 2001).

AIDS in the Workplace

The risk of contracting AIDS in the workplace is threefold, depending on occupation, work setting, and status (Akeroyd 2004). The risk of HIV transmission is inherent or integral to occupations that put workers in contact with blood and bodily fluids (all work in medicine and dentistry and all sex work, voluntary or coerced, including in tourism, entertainment, and domestic service). Risk is integral to dangerous occupations in which the rate of accidents and injuries is high, exposing workers to contaminated blood (military service, mining, industrial jobs, trucking, policing, and prison work). Risk is also high for migrant workers separated from family, for those who regularly travel long distances, and for personnel posted overseas (seasonal farm-workers, seafarers, airline crew, the military). Every work setting is risky in conflict zones.

Everything said above about sexism, racism, and class prejudice in the workplace compounds women's risk of contracting AIDS at work. Unequal gender relations, compounded by racial and ethnic hierarchies and by class and caste orders, conspire to place women at higher risk of infection in work settings. Everything discussed in chapter 5 about the sexual politics of violence against women amplifies women's chances of contracting AIDS at work. Sexual intercourse forced upon women and girls as part of interpersonal and institutional violence raises the risk. Economic and systemic violence that makes women dependent upon men for their livelihood, increases women's vulnerability to AIDS. Political violence that denies full citizenship to women, deprives women of protection against sexual harassment at work—what Akeroyd (2004) calls the sexualization of work environments.

Thirty years into the AIDS pandemic, the lack of information about which jobs pose greater risk, which work settings are especially hazardous, and how status—whether the high status of women in politics or the low status of girls in factories—affects risk, is egregious. Almost everywhere economic restructuring and global transformation are reinforcing preexisting inequalities and exclusions, such as sexism, racism, ethnic discrimination, and religious conflict (Parker and Aggleton 2003), yet the impact of these forces on women at work is poorly understood, and the relation of restructured economies to AIDS rarely investigated.

CHAPTER FOUR

Fighting for Good Health Services, Struggling with the Pharmaceutical Industry

The United Nations defines the right to health as the right to an effective and integrated health system that is responsive to national and local priorities, accessible to all, and encompasses health care and the underlying determinants of health (Commission on Human Rights 2006). The underlying determinants include adequate sanitation, safe drinking water, and health education as well as the social determinants of health, which are conditions like poverty and unemployment, parts of why people fall ill. An effective health system is a core social institution, no less than a court system or a political system. But the UN Special Rapporteur on the right to health carefully avoids discussion of whether this system should be publicly or privately financed (Commission on Human Rights 2006).

Health policy is a key public space for constraining and contesting inequality and exclusion. For women's health movements in the South, a critical moment arrived when they took the idea of women's right to control their fertility, which women's groups in the West had introduced in the 1970s, and incorporated it into a much broader vision that encompassed all of women's health needs (UNRISD 2000). Women's groups in the South saw that health care systems can embed and reinforce inequality within societies. They saw, too, that they could use health care systems to combat poverty and inequality by linking women's health rights to development. Many women's health groups have joined some of the larger health movement organizations like Medact, WEMOS, the People's Health Movement, and the International People's Health Council.[1]

The debates women's groups encounter when engaging the struggle for equitable health care systems are about whether governments or individuals are responsible for health and whether the public or private sector (or some public-private partnership) should provide health services. Government responsibility for health care was a prime demand during the decolonization of the global South; people saw the state as the only source of sufficient resources to meet the health needs of entire populations. Liberation movements also understood that public health services are emblematic of a regime's concern for its people and that building a health service for everyone legitimizes a government's claim to social justice. The converse is also true: inequitable and expensive health care impoverishes those on low incomes and reinforces social inequality (Mackintosh 2003).

Engaging the struggle for equitable health care systems brings women into direct confrontation with the multinational corporations and international institutions that have transformed health care in the past 20 years, commercializing both supply and expenditure. Women's groups are especially critical of the multinational pharmaceutical industry, and women's health movements have responded vigorously to breaches of ethics in medical research and clinical drug trials.

In the poorest countries, international development agencies have been pressing governments to turn the provision of health services over to charities and individual private practitioners as part of the regressive pattern of commercialization (Turshen 1999). In middle-income countries, the introduction of commercial health insurance moves systems toward more private profit seeking and reduced regulation. The effect of shifting from a tax-based system to one that charges a flat rate or variable fees for service is to exclude low-income users (Mackintosh 2003). The specific mix of public and private care and the configuration of each nation's system remain in flux as the World Bank continues to experiment in the vast laboratory that is the global South and as the corporatization of the health sector catches up. To achieve equality, women's groups work to block health care commodification and individual health insurance schemes; they have learned that it is not enough to demand regulation of the private sector.

The objective of this chapter is to show how women have suffered from the commercialization of both health care and health policy associated with globalization (discussed in chapter 2), and how women's groups have contested and tried to change the worldwide trends that have marked the provision of health care since the 1970s. The emphasis in the first part is on the key dimensions of health services that determine the extent of equity: access, cost, and the range and quality of services available to women of different classes, races, or other social groupings.

In addition to the basic issue of primary health care provision, the chapter also deals briefly with the specific problems of health services under difficult conditions—in wartime and in prison. The pharmaceutical industry and issues of research on women's health comprise the focus of the second part of the chapter.

Primary Health Care

Women and men do not participate equally in health care, either as users of health services (women use more) or as providers of health care (women provide more). Yet most health service systems cater to men and neglect women. Even when providers design services to meet women's needs, they often use male perspectives that are unresponsive to women's expectations or specific concerns. More health care, perhaps three-fourths, takes place at household or community level than in the formal health sector, and women provide most of that care. The reliance on women's unpaid care work in the household strains poor women already burdened with too many responsibilities and supported with too few resources. Women are community health workers and traditional birth attendants. They fill a high percentage of lower-level professional and ancillary staff positions in formal health services. The viability of primary health care services that are frequently under-resourced, often depends upon female health workers whose task is to support and work with the community. The health sector reforms currently underway in many countries will transform the structure of staffing as well as the incentives, skills, and rewards at various levels of the health system. Cuts in health and social sectors lead to higher levels of unemployment among women health workers, as well as increases in the work burdens of informal home care. These changes reinforce gender divisions of labor and gender biases in the provision of health care (Oxaal with Cook 1998).

A coalition of groups united under the banner of the Women's Global Network for Reproductive Rights demands, "Health for All Women, Health for All Now!" In the face of destructive reforms they are revising WHO's 1975 slogan, "Health for All by the Year 2000," which was the World Health Organization's unrealized promise of universal primary health care, and they are underscoring the importance of women's needs. Women's health movements have drawn our attention to the particular impact of private health care on women's access to services, and they have deplored the way that state health policies have compromised women's health. Although governments and international development institutions promote women's health in their rhetoric, they rarely take responsibility for women's compromised health. The World Bank strategy to impose user fees for public services, reinforced by international donors' practice of making user fees a condition of loans and aid, is now entrenched in many developing countries. These fees, coupled with the increase in private medical practice and an explosive growth in private pharmacies, reinforce gender inequality (UNRISD 2000). Rises in out-of-pocket costs for public and private health care services are driving many families into poverty and are increasing the poverty of those who are already poor, creating the situation known as "the medical poverty trap" (Whitehead, Dahlgren, and Evans 2001). Health sector reforms have not resolved the problems of providing uncontroversial services like maternal and child health services and family planning for married women, let alone controversial services like abortion and family planning for adolescents and unmarried women.

A renewed push for primary health care comes from the international agencies that are creating a two-tiered system (private care for the wealthy and public care for the poor) that is narrowly concerned only with women's reproductive health. The agencies' agreement to cloak reproductive issues in "women's reproductive rights" has not mollified women's health movements in countries like India. Indian women's groups, critical of the Beijing Platform for Action, note that obstetrical causes account for only 25 percent of all women's deaths; far more significant are the 65 percent of deaths caused by disease, predominantly infectious diseases (WGNRR 1995). The only disease named in the Beijing Platform is AIDS, but even in this case the document does not question the link between AIDS and poor health service systems. In contrast, the 1978 WHO/UNICEF Declaration of Alma Ata designed primary health care to address all health issues, including women's reproductive health needs and sexually transmitted infections. The demands of the Rural Women's Liberation Movement in Arakkonam, Tamil Nadu, India, protesting government plans to hand over primary health centers to the private sector, are direct: in order to safeguard motherhood and to provide adequate nutritional support to pregnant women, primary health centers should serve women's basic health needs and reduce deaths during delivery (WGNRR 2003f).

Accessibility

The Beijing Platform of Action did not address issues of accessibility of care, so important to the poor in rural and urban areas, according to the

Indian women's movement (WGNRR 1995). Women's groups believe that economic factors like the feminization of poverty determine accessibility even more than the physical availability of services. They see women's poverty as increasing the gaps between classes and affecting women's access to health care.

Countries with serious economic difficulties are not the only ones to record untreated sickness among poor people. Some nations with high and stable economic growth rates like China, formerly renowned for access to essential health services in rural areas, have drastically reduced accessibility. Despite a yearly economic growth rate of almost 10 percent in the past two decades, 35 to 40 percent of rural Chinese households report an illness for which they did not seek health care citing financial difficulties as the main reason. In addition, 60 percent of Chinese referred to hospital by a doctor never contacted the hospital because they knew they could not afford to pay the high user charges (Whitehead, Dahlgren, and Evans 2001).

High user fees typically cause an indiscriminate reduction in access to care. Justified as a measure to raise revenue from local people, user fees are "most ill advised" (UNRISD 2000). One study of 39 developing countries found that user fees increased revenues only slightly, while significantly reducing the access of low-income people to basic social services. Financial constraints cause poor people to delay seeking care at a health center until an emergency arises, which then forces them into more expensive care at a hospital. The negative effects of user fees are poorer health and increased medical expenditure, making the charges both inefficient and inequitable (Whitehead, Dahlgren, and Evans 2001).

The Asia-Pacific Resource and Research Center for Women (ARROW) reviewed seven Southeast Asian countries and found no increase in availability, accessibility, or affordability of primary health services in the 1990s. In fact, the costs of childbirth, medication, and reproductive health services increased with the introduction of user fees as part of privatization, health sector reform, and globalization. Reproductive health services remain less accessible to poor, migrant, and indigenous women and are largely unavailable for unmarried, young, and older women. Only in Malaysia and Thailand are primary health care services available to most of the population. "Governments have been unable to increase their budget for primary health care, especially due to the financial crisis of the late 1990s and less funding priority is given to the health sector" (Abdullah 2003, 34).

Government investments in education and health services are cornerstones of socioeconomic development. When public services are available and accessible, health indicators improve. In South Asia, the main public health challenge is the desperate state of maternal and child health: the neglect of mothers and children is driving the region's high morbidity and mortality rates (Bhutta, Nundy, and Abbasi 2004). Sri Lanka and the Indian state of Kerala show how it is possible to improve the situation. Despite a civil war, Sri Lanka has the best health indicators in the region (better than those of most other countries with comparable incomes), with average life expectancy at 73 years, infant mortality at 16 per 1,000 live births, and maternal mortality at 30 per 100,000 live births. The Indian state of Kerala has levels similar to Sri Lanka, achieving health and demographic indicators far ahead of Indian national averages; over 80 percent of infants in Kerala receive all routine vaccines in the first year of life, use of family planning services is high, and population growth is steady at replacement levels. Underpinning health and education investment strategies in both Kerala and Sri Lanka are a combination of political will and grassroots support. The keys to outstanding health and economic indicators for women are policies to achieve gender and social equity.

The problems of access are not limited to the geographical South. Women in Black (Belgrade), a chapter of an international antiwar group, complained at a one-day meeting they organized together with the Autonomous Women's Centre Against Sexual Violence in 2002 about increasing corruption in the health service sector, which they say necessitates the enforcement of laws to protect the dignity of both patients and medical staff. Health has become a consumer commodity instead of being a fundamental human right as it should be. Those who have more money have more health care (WGNRR 2003g).

Quality of Care

Quality of care relates closely to accessibility because access is not only a financial issue. In addition to chronic underfunding of public health services, lack of supplies and equipment, widespread use of informal "under-the-table" payments, and indirect costs of service use like transportation and loss of income, the ways staff treat patients also cause underuse. The failure to respect and respond to disadvantaged groups is an issue of quality of care. Women commonly acknowledge that health professionals are rude to them. Many women complain of insults and ill treatment, even of being beaten, and they resent the lack of privacy and confidentiality; the hostile atmosphere causes them to hesitate about asking questions about options and available services. Hierarchies of education, class, caste, and, in some countries, race, and ethnicity mar the relationship between women and health practitioners.

Health care providers routinely neglect adolescents as a group. In Nigeria, health workers subject girls to unfriendly treatment and inappropriate care, sometimes failing to protect the confidentiality of sensitive medical records, involving reproductive health, unwanted pregnancies, and sexually transmitted diseases (Madunagu 2001). Typically, young people treated in this way resort to the services of herbalists, fall into the hands of quacks, or simply try to self-medicate. The Nigerian Coalition for Youth Friendly Health Services and the Girl Power Initiative held a sensitization workshop on the problems in Calabar in 2001.

The Women's Health Project of South Africa (www.wits.ac.za/whp accessed 25 July 2006) documented the concerns that service users have: first and foremost is how providers treat patients. Second on the list was the time patients have to wait for service and the need to come back on different days for different services. Then came issues such as poor drug supplies, inadequate resources, and the desire for additional services, specifically increased access around the clock. The Women's Health Project believes that addressing these issues requires improving the way the entire health system functions, for which a health systems approach is essential. The task is to improve the quality of the existing services, take the staff who work in the system seriously, and then move on to increasing the range of services. The piecemeal, single-issue focus that characterizes much of the work in reproductive health care nationally and internationally allows researchers, NGOs, and governments to continue as before, maintaining their narrow specialist interests or services. Health Workers for Change, an intervention to improve the environment in health care facilities, unearthed health systems issues as the preeminent causes for poor quality of care. The Health Workers for Change program creates a positive attitude among staff who recommit themselves to their work in spite of frustrations. It also sets out the roles and responsibilities that managers must fulfill to support health care providers in maintaining caring services.

The adequacy of management to health system functioning is possibly the center of this big challenge. Rather than beginning with the discourse of integrated services, the Women's Health Project began with the day-to-day reality of service provision, making the rhetoric of integrated primary health care a reality. In South Africa's Northern Province, an integration project encouraged staff to describe, analyze, and resolve their own problems. The project resulted in improved drug ordering and reorganization: some local staff decided to move from overstaffed to understaffed clinics, increasing equity. Daily routines changed: staff provided all services in one room on one day, meeting patient needs and also increasing job satisfaction. Staff do resist and challenge such changes, which can occur nonetheless.

Like the Women's Health Project, the Bangladesh Women's Health Coalition believes that positive treatment of patients begins with positive treatment of staff. Good managers give staff a voice in making decisions and treat staff with respect; staff, in turn, interact positively with patients. Participatory management style encourages responsiveness to and communication with patients, and both are essential to the provision of quality health care services (Kay, Germain, and Bangser 1991).

Quality of care expressed in satisfaction with respectful treatment motivates some women to seek out traditional healers.

Traditional Health Care

Any discussion of traditional health care begins by recognizing the colonial state's role, abetted by Christian medical missionaries, in determining the growth and development (or stagnation and corruption) of indigenous practices. In some countries missionaries were the advance guard of the colonists, and they confused traditional religious ceremonies with traditional health care, devaluing both which they regarded as in competition with their proselytism. The record of governments is more mixed.

Other colonial governments banned or suppressed traditional healers, leaving women fewer options and in the long term depriving traditional healers of biomedical knowledge that might have enhanced their skills. Attitudes changed in the postcolonial era. WHO and many governments began to regard traditional healers as allies who could complement biomedical care, or even—in the case of mental illness—provide more effective care. In the global South women's illiteracy and the even greater class gulf between physician and patient complicate the problems of uninformative treatment. Because biomedical health providers tend to make women in the South feel incompetent, it is not surprising that patients prefer traditional healers who may explain their illnesses. Whereas biomedical practitioners give limited information and instruct women on what to do, traditional healers often help make sense of illness, explaining the problem and telling patients what they can do in the future to avoid sickness. Women are seeking global interpretations that refer to their beliefs and representations, rather than reasons for illness based on scientific discourse (De Koninck 1998). Pregnant poor women may be more inclined to consult traditional birth attendants because they are culturally sensitive, respectful, and cost less than mainstream health services.

In some countries, thriving local midwifery practices provided obstetric care, contraception, and abortion. When Third World governments invited European medical doctors to take charge, they displaced local practitioners. In Egypt, the modernizing state of Muhammad 'Ali (1805–1848) invited the French physician Antoine Barthelme Clot to organize a hospital, a medical school, and a school of midwifery (Hatem 2000). Clot's aim was to substitute a new professional group of educated midwives whom the principles of modern medicine would guide; above all, he wanted to put an end to abortion. In the process, he removed women's autonomy and suppressed their wishes, needs, and desires (Hatem 2000). Registration of births and deaths enforced the new police powers of public health workers by enabling them to keep track of family life.

Many developing countries now offer a variety of medical services with choices ranging from government, mission, and private biomedical facilities and commercial drug outlets to traditional private practitioners and traditional pharmacists (Tipping and Segall 1995). In Benin, Indonesia, and Mali, traditional practitioners are popular because they cost less and are more flexible about arrangements for payment than commercial pharmacies (Oxaal with Cook 1998). Women in poor households may use home remedies or consult traditional pharmacists before turning to commercial pharmacies for drugs sold without a prescription.

An innovative group of traditional healers and doctors in Uganda formed THETA (Traditional and Modern Health Practitioners Together against AIDS) in 1990 to evaluate the effectiveness of herbal medicine for AIDS-related chronic wasting, chronic diarrhea, and Herpes Zoster as alternatives to unavailable biomedical treatments. Another initiative of the project is THEWA (Traditional Healers, Women and AIDS Prevention), which developed a gender-sensitive, culturally appropriate strategy for educating and counseling people on HIV and AIDS (Butcher and Welbourn 2001).

The infiltration of discriminatory gender attitudes into medical knowledge is not a Western monopoly. Traditional medical systems may accept discriminatory gender norms just as biomedicine does. For example, in the highlands of Peru people believe that wind or air-borne factors related to the supernatural environment are the principal causes of sickness. Because women have a more "open" physiology than men and because they lose bodily fluids and blood during menstruation and pregnancy, highlanders consider women to be disadvantaged and weak. Because of these "handicaps" they restrict women from engaging in hard work and from traveling to the lowlands where the cash economy and the lucrative gold mining industry are located; at the same time they devalue women's domestic work as being light work (Sen, George, and Östlin 2002).

Health Services in Wartime

War and imprisonment are two special circumstances in which women's health care choices are even more limited than usual and in which their vulnerability and need for care are heightened. For women caught up in war, even traditional healers may not be available. Military-imposed curfews, sieges, and refugee camps are routine in warfare that escalates already unmet needs and creates new ones. How to provide medical care when the existing government and private hospitals are already insufficient and rebels kidnap doctors or the government armed forces conscript them? When rebel forces target clinics and health workers for destruction? How to provide health education and medical training when war closes or destroys schools, children are in hiding with their families, or fleeing to camps, or rebels capture and force them to serve in their armies?

In Palestine, at the beginning of the first *intifada* that started in 1987, responsibility for finding solutions to problems like these fell to the women. "Organized on neighborhood, district, city-wide, regional and national levels, the women's committees had for years played a critical role in . . . the nationalist movement" (Bennis 1990, 31). The Union of Palestinian Women's Committees, the Palestinian Working Women's Committee, the Women's Committee for Social Work, the Women's Action Committee in Dheisha refugee camp have all mobilized to work harder, handle more cases, and take on new roles. Better able to move around during curfews than men, women obtain food and supplies, storing large amounts at home; and they organize food production and preparation for long sieges when the Israeli Defense Force blocks any movement in or out of villages and camps. The Society of In'ash el-Usra, a charity run by women, is helping four times the number of people as before the first *intifada*; it is selling women's embroidery and collecting clothes for prisoners to be distributed through the Red Crescent.

Medical care provided by the various Palestinian medical organizations is coordinated by the women's associations: they conduct first-aid training, mobilize blood donations and blood-typing campaigns, and smuggle medical personnel into closed areas to treat the wounded. Popular education, the alternative (and illegal) classes designed to circumvent the forced closing of the schools, is implemented by separated neighborhood committees, but coordinated by the women's groups (Bennis 1990, 32).

During the first year of the *intifada*, over 35,000 people, mostly young women, were trained in emergency care—a rigorous course of 20 sessions on how to deal with fractures, gas inhalation, cardiac arrest, and other critical conditions (Bennis 1990). The blood-typing campaigns involve registering potential blood donors and listing their blood types at neighborhood, regional, and central levels so that transfusions for gunshot victims can be made without delay. Women make up 90 percent of villagers needing primary health care, and women doctors are needed to treat them, but in 2003, according to the Medical Association Registry, only 22 (16 percent) out of 137 registered obstetricians were female (www.wclac.org/reports/health.html accessed 15 September 2006).

Medical Treatment in Women's Prisons

The inadequacies of women's medical care in prison appear to be universal, as reports from Great Britain, Lebanon, Pakistan, Peru, South Korea, the United States, and other countries attest. This failure is unsurprising as a military design for healthy young men is the basis of the system (Cooper 2002). This section is limited to the problems of prison medical care (see chapter 5 for a discussion of the abuse of women prisoners).[2]

The British women's movements brought pressure on authorities to reform women's prisons in the 1960s. The British government planned to redesign Holloway, the most important prison for women, to operate as a secure hospital on the assumption that most women and girls in custody require some form of medical, psychiatric, or remedial treatment; in the end it built special facilities only for mentally disturbed prisoners (Zedner 1995).

In the four women's prisons in Lebanon, conditions may amount to cruel, inhuman, and degrading treatment (Amnesty International 2001). The government is not attending adequately to the medical needs of a large number of sick prisoners and is holding them in conditions falling short of Lebanese law and the UN Standard Minimum Rules. Hygienic and sanitary conditions in these institutions are seriously inadequate. Dormitories are overcrowded, damp, poorly ventilated, and infested by vermin. Visitors report that authorities lock up detainees most of the time and allow no access to fresh air or exercise. The women have no beds and sleep on the floor using foam mattresses.

Jail conditions are notorious in Pakistan; women and children mix with the adult male prison population, and little or no women's health care is available. The organization Lawyers for Human Rights and Legal Aid (LHRLA) has been active in bringing about much-needed jail reforms in the country (www.lhrla.sdnpk.org/reforms.html accessed 15 September 2006). In 1992 the group challenged the presence of women prisoners in Karachi Central jail, fought against illegal detentions, and torture, and LHRLA succeeded in gaining a separate prison for women, a dispensary in the women's jail, the first-ever female superintendent of women's jails, and legal aid for prisoners.

The world learned of the treatment of women prisoners in Peru after the conviction of Lori Berenson, a U.S. citizen. A political prisoner, authorities sent her to the infamous Yanamayo prison, located in a remote region of the Peruvian Andes at an altitude of over 12,000 feet above sea level, where she suffered from serious medical problems. Conditions in Yanamayo and Challapalca prisons are so harsh that they amount to cruel, inhuman, or degrading treatment according to the Inter-American Commission on Human Rights. The inaccessibility of the prisons seriously limits prisoners' rights to maintain contact with the outside world, including relatives, lawyers, and doctors. Political prisoners in several high-security prisons throughout Peru have staged protests, including hunger strikes, calling for an improvement in prison conditions (Nottingham 2004).

The prison system in South Korea also does not conform to international standards as it lacks medical facilities and care, restricts exercise, uses solitary confinement, lacks heating in winter, and inflicts punishments on prisoners (Amnesty International 1998). Both male and female prisoners are at risk, but women prisoners have special health needs for which there is no provision. Women in Chongju Prison, the only women's prison, report difficulties obtaining sanitary items. Authorities invariably hold women political prisoners in solitary confinement with little or no human contact.

In the United States, women make up only 8.4 percent of 1.93 million prisoners; authorities often overlook their special medical needs—from gynecological problems to histories of sexual and physical abuse (94 percent of incarcerated women have such pasts). Prisons fail in prevention, screening, diagnosis, treatment, continuity of care, alleviation of pain, rehabilitation, and recovery from reproductive and breast cancers. A 1997 Bureau of Justice study found that 30 percent of women in federal facilities reported a medical problem, compared with 23 percent of men.

In 1999, Amnesty International documented egregious violations of women's general medical care. Access to a doctor is often conditional on permission by nonmedical staff, who may underestimate the seriousness of the case or refuse to believe inmates. When authorities do respond to emergencies, they often use handcuffs and shackles on women during transport and in hospital, even if they do not have a history of violence or escape; using restraints poses a serious health threat to women giving birth. Many women experiencing mental problems routinely receive psychotropic drugs because other forms of more appropriate treatment such as counseling or psychotherapy are unavailable. A U.S. Justice Department investigation into Julia Tutwiler prison for women in Alabama concluded in 1995 that the prison's mental health care program was almost inexistent (Amnesty International 1999). The federal government refuses Medicaid payments for prisoners, placing the entire burden on states. Nor does the federal government hold the prison medical system, which is uncoordinated and underfunded, accountable. Doctors are ill trained and overburdened and correctional personnel can overrule their decisions. Some states contract out to private corporations: Correctional Medical Services (www.cmsstl.com) has contracts with more than 300 prisons and jails in 31 states including an $89 million contract for New Jersey's correctional health care (Cooper 2002).

Women and the Pharmaceutical Industry

Broad general problems link the pharmaceutical industry to the uneven delivery of health services in the global South. Pharmaceutical prices drive health care budgets in the global South, accounting for 10 to 40 percent of public health budgets and 20 to 50 percent of total health care expenditures (Murray, Govindaraj, and Chellaraj 1994); in Mali the total figure was an astounding 66 percent (Coulibaly and Keita 1993). The comparable figure for the United States is 12 percent of total health care expenditures. Pharmaceuticals are so important in the global South because, in the absence of adequate numbers of trained health personnel, basic drugs given according to standardized regimens can stretch limited health budgets to cover many more people.

Industry Practices

Health budgets would stretch further if drugs were less expensive, and one way to reduce prices is to manufacture drugs locally instead of importing them from multinational companies. Few countries in the global South have the facilities to manufacture pharmaceuticals, and the World Bank actively discourages countries from developing them on the grounds that such efforts would be inefficient and wasteful of scarce resources (World Bank 1993). India set up a self-reliant drug industry, with Soviet help, in 1961, creating the Indian public sector to produce vital drugs; private sector investment followed and, with a government policy restricting multinational industry in the late 1970s, India became capable of producing most essential drugs. As a result, antibiotic prices fell by 60 or 70 percent (Gupta 1999). Eventually, in the mid-1980s the multinationals beat back the Indian restrictions, as liberalization swept the country. By 2005, India had joined the WTO (World Trade Organization) and agreed to abide by international patent regulations. Not every country can imitate the Indian success, but Zimbabwe tried and might have succeeded had the World Bank helped instead of actively undermining the local industry (Turshen 1999).

Generics are another answer to high priced brand name drugs, and Big Pharma (the colloquial name for the industry) has fought their introduction, systematically creating "branded generics" and claiming that the brand stands for quality control. Branded generics have profit margins of 70 percent, twice that of regular generics. The multinationals routinely sue small companies trying to manufacture generic versions of their drugs, claiming patent infringement. Even if they lose the lawsuit, they have successfully delayed production (which under law cannot go forward while the lawsuit is outstanding) and reaped the additional profits of monopoly protection.

Patents, which grant monopoly protection for 20 years, sustain the system of high prices and high profits. Free trade agreements protect patent rights, limiting access to medications. Trade agreements like TRIPS (Trade-Related Aspects of Intellectual Property Rights), implemented through the World Intellectual Property Organization (WIPO), restrict access to the most needed medications under patent (Onori 2006; PANOS 2002). Despite all the industry's arguments, the adverse effect of patents on the availability of medicines has led to public outrage, as well as explicit recommendations for changes in WTO and WIPO patent procedures (Waitzkin 2003).

The pharmaceutical industry is relentless in its pursuit of profits, blocking every measure agencies take to rein in its practices, as the following examples attest. When WHO, prompted by groups like INFACT and the Baby Food Action Group, demanded a code of conduct for the sale of infant formula, President Ronald Reagan instructed the U.S. delegation to the 1981 World Health Assembly to vote against it (and the U.S. delegate, Dr Steve Jonas, resigned rather than cast a "no" vote). U.S. firms, backed by the U.S. government, blocked the development of an international code of conduct for pharmaceutical manufacturers. The International Federation of Pharmaceutical Manufacturers Associations (IFPMA), representing the industry in 47 countries, promoted its own code of pharmaceutical manufacturing practice, which is so loosely worded that it serves only to legitimize existing unacceptable standards of promotion in developing countries (Melrose 1982). During President Bill Clinton's administration, pharmaceutical companies sued the government of South Africa for trying to import cheap drugs to treat AIDS. Manufacturers blocked the government of Bangladesh, one of the poorest countries in the world, from adopting WHO's recommended policy of limiting the national formulary to 200 essential drugs; the companies threatened to boycott and sanction Bangladesh, mainly by denying other needed drugs and products (Koehler 2006).

Health movements, including groups like Health Action International[3] and women's health movements, do not level the accusation of rapacious practices against the pharmaceutical industry lightly. Study after study has documented corporate greed. From the U.S. Congressional hearings that Senator Estes Kefauver held from 1959–1961, to the research of the UN Conference on Trade and Development (UNCTAD) in the 1960s, and the U.K. Monopolies Commission investigations of the industry in the 1970s, the record is unambiguous. Pharmaceutical companies are extortionate—and lucrative. Combined profits for the 10 drug companies in the Fortune 500 ($35.9 billion in 2002) were more than the profits for all the other 490 businesses put together ($33.7 billion); put another way, yearly pharmaceutical industry profits of 18.5 percent are well above the median 4.6 percent for all industries (Angell 2004). To protect profits, Big Pharma spent $60 million lobbying the U.S. Congress in 1999—more than any other industry including insurance, tobacco, utilities, oil and gas. The top 40 U.S. pharmaceutical companies spent more than $5.3 billion in 1998 to employ 56,000 people to push their products and another $1 billion on marketing events for doctors.

Total worldwide sales for prescription drugs were about $400 billion in 2002 (about half were in the United States, the major profit center), but this figure underestimates real spending because it does not include drugs administered in hospitals, nursing homes, or doctors' offices (Angell 2004). The market for drugs that treat diseases and conditions specific to women, including breast, uterine, and ovarian cancers, menopause, fertility, and infertility, reached $5.7 billion in sales in 1995; that figure was growing at a compound annual rate of 19 percent and analysts projected it would top $10.6 billion in 2000 (Key and Marble 1996). This figure underestimates women's consumption of drugs, especially because the elderly constitute the largest market for medicines in the industrial countries and, with longer life expectancies, women outnumber men in this age group.

Irrational prescribing and drug resistance make an important, but overlooked, contribution to the inequities of the medical poverty trap (Whitehead, Dahlgren, and Evans 2001). Irrational prescription includes overprescribing (people are taking many more drugs than they used to) and the prescription of new more expensive drugs instead of older, cheaper ones. The industry adds to these problems by routinely raising the prices of the most heavily prescribed drugs, sometimes several times a year (Angell 2004). In India, 52 percent of out-of-pocket health expenditure went toward medicines and fees, as did 71 percent of in-patient expenditure (Iyer and Sen 2000).

The industry argues that prices are high because research and development are costly. But research and development are relatively small parts of the budgets of the big drug companies. In the 1990s, roughly 36 percent of sales went into marketing and administration, a poorly defined category that includes advertising, promotion, education, legal costs, and executive salaries (salaries are no small item: the CEO of Bristol-Myers-Squibb made $75 million in salary and $76 million in stock options in 2001). Marketing and administration accounted for two and a half times as much as research and development (Angell 2004).

The pharmaceutical industry spends billions on corporate image portraying humanitarianism as its motivation to cut the rate of profit through voluntary reductions to the lowest viable commercial price. Price cuts and drug donation programs (which come with tax advantages) are not so spontaneous or voluntary. Organized professionals, nonprofessional health workers, activists, and governments struggle with corporations to reduce prices and donate medications (Waitzkin 2003).

A second counter argument to the industry's defense of its prices is that the public sector pays for 30 percent of research and development. Moreover, most research and development dollars go toward mimicking successful products of rival firms or to lifestyle drugs like Viagra. Companies peg prices at what the market will bear; manufacturing accounts for only 40 percent of total costs.

A company typically tests a new drug on animals and, if it is promising with no disqualifying adverse effects, physicians will conduct clinical trials at the company's request and publish the results in medical journals. These articles then become part of the company's submission to the government agency that approves drugs for the market. Women complain that physicians, especially in the global South, do not record or take seriously the secondary effects they report. Now the American Medical Association, joined by a group of leading medical publications, has adopted a resolution urging the federal government to create a database to register all trials performed in the United States (Meier 2004a). They are concerned that drug industry sponsorship of such tests affects the quality of medical practice. Companies that sponsor the trials and the medical journals that publish the reports tend to spotlight positive findings and suppress negative or inconclusive results; and the companies submit different parts of tests under different authors' names to different medical journals for maximum publicity (Meier 2004b). The drug industry has effectively turned journals into a marketing arm, even though medical editors require authors to disclose financial ties to the drug's marketer (Meier 2004b). As expected, PhRMA (the Pharmaceutical Research and Manufacturers Association of America, the powerful industry trade association) does not support the creation of such a registry.

Another strategy is to market diseases rather than drugs by campaigning to create awareness of the affliction and by inventing new conditions or false needs for which companies also create the treatment or cure (Sample 2006). For example, drug firms have created campaigns to raise awareness of generalized anxiety disorder (GAD), with symptoms of restlessness, fatigue, irritability, muscle tension, nausea, diarrhea, and sweating, which they say afflicts as many as ten million Americans with paralyzing irrational fears (Koerner 2002). To treat this new disease, GlaxoSmithKline, which had developed the antidepressant Paxil in 1993, asked the U.S. Food and Drug Administration (FDA) to approve its use in the treatment of generalized anxiety disorder. In 2001 on the date of approval of FDA, a patient group called Freedom from Fear released a telephone survey that found people with GAD spent nearly 40 hours per week, the equivalent of a full-time job, worrying. GlaxoSmithKline's public relations firm sponsored the survey (Koerner 2002). Thus, in one campaign GlaxoSmithKline accomplished two aims: it prolonged and expanded the use of a very profitable drug.

A recent trend in the pharmaceutical industry is to use for-profit research organizations instead of universities to develop new drugs (Rothman 2000). Between 1991 and 2000, the percent of pharmaceutical industry funding for clinical trials in academic medical centers dropped from 80 to 50 percent (Bodenheimer 2000). Pharmaceutical companies are contracting with research organizations to speed up the process, reduce the costs of drug testing, and shorten the time between the discovery and marketing of new drugs. At universities, researchers must apply to institutional review boards and human subject committees; contract research organizations can bypass these ethical checkpoints, saving time and the added cost of redesigning studies to meet ethical standards. The implications for Third World women who are frequently the subjects of clinical trials are disturbing.

Women Push Back

Women are potential beneficiaries of the multinational pharmaceutical industry's products, but too often they have been the victims of its negligent practices. The media have exposed some of the problems women experience at the hands of the pharmaceutical industry: DES, the early formulations of the contraceptive pill, thalidomide, the Dalkon shield, and bromocriptine all caused severe health problems and some women died. In each case, doctors prescribed the drug to improve reproductive health, but the results were devastating. This section briefly recaps each of these cases in turn.

Doctors began prescribing diethylstilbestrol (DES) in the 1940s to prevent miscarriage; nearly six million American women ingested the drug between 1943 and 1959 (Marks 2001). Twenty years later their daughters developed vaginal cancer (an extremely rare disease) and their sons were born with undescended testicles or they developed cysts in the urogenital system (WHO 2003a). The California-based Coalition for the Medical Rights of Women[4] founded DES Action in 1976; they urged the state health department to alert women and doctors to the dangers of DES. DES Action continues today as an independent national organization (www.desaction.org).

Although doctors in Great Britain reported thromboembolisms in women using the contraceptive pill in 1961—one year after GD Searle first marketed the hormonal combination—nearly a decade passed before the manufacturer admitted problems; pills containing high doses of estrogen remained on sale until the U.K. government forced their withdrawal in December 1969 (Marks 2001). Researchers first reported the link between the pill and cancer in 1964, but they found the tumors in rats, and the pharmaceutical and chemical industries have long resisted the extrapolation of animal studies to humans. The long gestation period (15 to 25 years) for cancer meant that the industry could market the pill with impunity for the lifetime of the patent; for women, it meant elevated risk of developing breast and cervical cancers, the two most important cancers for women. In response to strong pressure from women's groups and a vigorous debate over the adequacy of drug information provided to patients, the U.S. government required manufacturers to insert warnings in the pill's packaging to alert women of the drug's adverse effects and dangers; such warning were to become a standard component in nearly all consumer packaging of drugs (Marks 2001).

Not until 1996 did researchers publish a comprehensive study concluding that death rates from breast cancer were higher among women who were using or had recently used the pill (women who had stopped more than 10 years before showed no excess mortality) (Marks 2001). Breast cancer is more common among higher income women who have had fewer or no pregnancies. Cervical cancer is more common among women in the global South, particularly among women who have given birth to many children, had many sexual partners, or whose partners were promiscuous (Paolisso and Leslie 1995). Long-term use of the pill (defined as five years or more) is causally associated with persistent human papilloma virus and cervical cancer (WHO 2002a). A two-fold increased cancer risk is potentially critical in the global South where women have many pregnancies, suffer untreated sexually transmitted diseases like human papilloma virus, are rarely screened for cervical cancer, and are subject to aggressive family planning programs marketing the pill.

Before the thalidomide scandal broke in 1962, the industry undertook no research on the effects of drugs prescribed during pregnancy. Thalidomide, a drug given to pregnant women to help them sleep better, caused babies to be born with flippers instead of arms and feet; the scandal resulted in major changes in the regulation of clinical trials of new pharmaceuticals (Sjöström and Nilsson 1972).

Another contraceptive scandal emerged in 1974: the Dalkon shield, an intrauterine device, caused uterine infection and sterility. Women's lawsuits moved the U.S. FDA to withdraw the device in 1975, and AH Robbins, the manufacturer, settled a class action lawsuit, closing the compensation trust only in April 2000. But Robbins continued to sell the Dalkon shield in the global South through 1989, with the aid of USAID (www.espi.com).

In the IUD case, women's lawsuits were effective, but in many other cases the pharmaceutical industry took no action, in part because they paid professionals to conduct clinical trials in societies that regularly ignore women's complaints so that serious adverse effects (routinely trivialized as side effects) were under-reported. It usually took considerable consumer pressure by groups like the Health Research Group led by Dr Sidney Wolfe before the U.S. FDA intervened. For example, the FDA took no action on the lactation suppression drug bromocriptine, which caused

32 deaths from strokes, seizures, heart attacks, and hypertension between 1980 and 1994, until 1995 when it was finally banned (www.nlm.nih.gov/medlineplus/druginfo/uspdi/202094.html accessed 21 March 2007).

Because the industry spends so much money on advertising and marketing directly to doctors and the public (U.S. manufacturers spent $1.85 billion in 1999 marketing directly to consumers), doctors are prone to overprescribe. In the 1950s and 1960s, doctors prescribed psychotropics (barbiturates and tranquillizers like the benzodiazepines Valium and Librium) for women's depression, without paying attention to subsequent problems of addiction or the psychosocial causes of their condition. Phyllis Chesler (1972) spearheaded women's opposition to the drugging of women dissatisfied with their lives in her path breaking study, *Women and Madness*. Advertisements for these drugs in the 1960s typically pictured a white male doctor's hand taking the pulse of a gray woman patient; the caption read, "whatever the diagnosis, prescribe Librium" (Women's Health Action Foundation 1995).

No serious research contested industry claims about the efficacy of hormone replacement therapy (HRT), although many doctors were aware that pharmaceutical companies manipulate women's fears, needs, and desires in order to make greater profits. The marketing of HRT played upon women's fear of growing old, promising that estrogen could delay the ageing process. Even after conclusive proof that estrogen causes cancer of the uterus in some women, the industry pushed a new formulation with all the sales experience of cosmetics marketers (Lumsden 2005). The National Women's Health Network testified before the U.S. FDA in 1991 that companies were promoting a potentially risky drug with the same techniques that the Publishers Clearinghouse Sweepstakes used (Worcester and Whatley 2000). Women's groups like the National Organization for Women (NOW) pressed for the Women's Health Initiative, one project of which was to undertake the first large-scale independent clinical trials of HRT. This study has disproved nearly every industry claim for HRT, showing that it does not protect women from heart attacks as claimed, does not protect against Alzheimer's disease, and does not protect against osteoporosis, that it causes breast cancer or raises the risks of the disease, that it increases the risk of strokes and blood clots, and increases risk of gall bladder disease (Notman and Nadelson 2002). Scientists are crediting the 50 percent drop in prescriptions of a popular HRT following the announcement of these findings in 2002 with the recent precipitous drop in breast cancer rates in the United States (see chapter 6 for more details).

The industry also routinely uses women in the global South as guinea pigs in clinical trials of new drugs. Women have encountered numerous problems with industry research trials: experimentation on women in clinical trials of new drugs; reckless disregard of women's safety; the fiction of informed consent; and the failure to follow up with participants. Manufacturers also fail to take responsibility for health problems connected to their products, claiming that patients misused products and shifting the blame to users (for more details see section on research below).

Women's health movements have been on the pharmaceutical industry's case since Barbara Seaman published *The Doctor's Case against the Pill* in 1969. GD Searle, one of the companies that sold the contraceptive pill, tried to suppress the book's publication, and leaders of family planning like Alan Guttmacher and Elizabeth Connell of Planned Parenthood criticized Seaman's thesis that the pill was dangerous, even deadly (Seaman 1995). Women fighting Big Pharma joined consumer movements to sue manufacturers for damaging products. Uniting with NGOs like INFACT, women's groups protested the failure to protect lactating women and their babies against unscrupulous infant formula sales practices around the world (www.stopcorporateabuse.org/cms/page1128.cfm accessed 21 March 2007).

Research on Women's Health

Researchers play an important role in defining women's health and in determining the issues that the medical establishment and the scientific world will regard as legitimate female health problems and which they will dismiss. Researchers, and those who fund research—industry, universities, and governmental agencies—determine which issues are eligible for research funding and, even more profoundly, how researchers will frame these questions. Will they see problems as biological, medical, social, political, economic, or cultural? The framing in turn dictates the choice of methodology. In the past, biomedical research systematically ignored the complex relationships of race, ethnicity, and health, failing to distinguish whether these characteristics are biological or societal attributes, and failing to study the intersection of these characteristics and their relationship to health (Narrigan et al. 1997).

Men dominate most research, as administrators, workers, and subjects. Some studies have a built-in male bias because they use data that do not accurately represent women's experiences; for example, studies using hospital or clinic records reflect the more frequent attendance of men and therefore under-represent women's health problems. Hospital and clinic records are poor sources of data for the most common diseases and causes of deaths among women; so are death certificates if doctors do not perform autopsies.

Profit is the focus of many studies, especially those by and for the pharmaceutical industry. The exclusion of one gender in clinical trials of new pharmaceuticals was categoric: researchers often denied women access to participation. As late as 2000, women accounted for only 12 percent of participants in clinical trials for drugs to treat AIDS. Pharmaceutical companies (often wrongly) generalize the results of research and clinical trials on men to women of varying ethnicities and ages they have not studied.

The failure of women to present themselves in sufficient numbers to allow analysis or draw significant conclusions is another reason researchers frequently give for the exclusion of women subjects from clinical trials. Based on past experiences of exploitation in high-risk clinical trials, women of color may decline participation. When the U.S. National Institutes of Health (NIH) receives funding for their research projects, apart from the projects of the Women's Health Initiative, they do not usually make women's health issues a priority. Pressure from the women's health movements caused the U.S. government to redress gender inequality in biomedical research by formally recognizing inequity in women's biomedical research in its 1985 report; and in 1990 NIH received a mandate to include women in all research grants. The Women's Health Initiative recruited women scientists to head at least 15 of 40 clinical centers. The NIH Reauthorization Act of 1993, which revised and extended NIH programs, required "blanket" inclusion of women in clinical studies and permanently established the Office of Research on Women's Health and the Office for Minority Health.

Even when studies include women, investigators may choose not to report differences or similarities by gender. The practice of assuming that the results of research on men can be applied to women can be detrimental to the health of women worldwide. For example, despite early recognition in the 1980s that AIDS was ravaging the health of women, investigators undertook little research on the different progression of the disease in women and men, on the opportunistic infections peculiar to women, or on the different challenges of managing them. Some research shows sex differences in length of survival, levels of viral load, and drug toxicity; women and men need different treatment with antiretroviral drugs and different management of opportunistic infections (Tallis 2002).

Researchers need to uncover the reasons underlying the unjust exclusion of women and to acknowledge the diversity of women, as well as their biological and social differences from men.

The lack of research on conditions significantly affecting low-income women and other groups (adolescents, older, disabled, rural, and urban women, women of color, and lesbians) reflects the inability of these groups to access quality healthcare (Narrigan et al. 1997). The lack of research is not exclusive to the United States; if anything the neglect of women's health is even greater in the global South. A survey of the literature on women's health research in Nigeria found that studies of women's reproductive health commenced only in the 1990s, even though family planning clinics started operating in the early 1970s (Adekanye 1999). The deficiency begins with the failure to collect data on women's health: when deaths occur at home, as they do in most of rural Africa, no one records the cause of death. Even when rural clinics exist, medical knowledge may be insufficient and laboratory facilities lacking to make an accurate diagnosis. Thus the tally of causes of death does not include women.

Some of the reasons that research is predominantly based on men are structural. First, the concepts of illness are gender based. Medicine categorizes diseases as women's or men's, and the lack of interest in women's diseases reflects the low status of women in society. Defining disease in this gendered way leads doctors to overlook certain conditions in women; for example, specialists associate lung cancer and coronary artery disease with men and they miss the symptoms in women because they do not manifest themselves in the same way as in men.

Second, individual scientists do not work on problems entirely of their own choosing: they carry out research to produce marketable results, which means publications, promotion, and peer recognition. Women's issues do not carry prestige in these markets. Even when researchers are interested in women's health, they may not receive support for their projects from private industry or government, which finance most research endeavors. The problem is greater in the global South. In South Africa, an audit of protocols submitted to the Medical Research Council (MRC) for short-term grants in 1996 showed that of 170 applications, men submitted 126, women 44; the MRC funded 70 percent of men's application's, accounting for 81.5 percent of all funds; they funded 22 percent of women's application's, accounting for 18.5 percent of the total (Hoosain, Jewkes, and Maphumalo 1998).

Third, women constitute a small proportion of scientists and research physicians. Almost exclusively, elite men conceptualize and construct health research questions. The boards that review research projects, control research funds, and decide who should study what and how have few women as administrators and scientific advisors. Some feminists believe that the scientific questions asked and answered depend more on who has the power to do the asking than on which biological or behavioral questions need answers (Narrigan et al. 1997). Investigators with a track record have the best chance of receiving funding and most women are still in the lower rungs of the hierarchy; few have accumulated extensive research records and they may find it necessary to work with a powerful mentor.

Finally, in times of budgetary pressure, funding goes to mainstream work, which is prejudicial to research on diseases important to women that may require new methodologies to explore new questions. Or funding goes to research on immediate technological solutions to problems, rather than finding environmental, behavioral, or risk factors to reduce the risk of disease. Pharmaceutical manufacturers and research entrepreneurs benefit from short-term approaches.

One rationalization for the intentional exclusion of women from biomedical research is that it is easier to record the experimental variable in homogeneous subjects. Such homogeneous research is less expensive to conduct and relatively more certain to yield significant results. Researchers regard women as deviations from male norms and believe that hormonal changes due to menstrual cycles, pregnancy, or lactation are problematic, not easily controlled, and likely to confound results. Furthermore, since the thalidomide debacle heightened sensitivity to teratogens, researchers fear that experimental treatments or interventions may harm the pregnant woman and her fetus creating legal liabilities. The U.S. FDA changed its guidelines to insist on women's participation in drug trials in 1997.[5]

Questions Needing Answers

A number of urgent questions about women's health need research. First, is there a sex-based biological difference in disease itself? The question is not whether a set of diseases specific to women differs from a set of diseases specific to men—obviously diseases specific to the reproductive organs are sex-specific. Nor is the question whether the diagnosis and treatment of women and men are different—plenty of studies show that they are. The question is, does the same disease manifest itself differently in men and women? Would sex-based biological differences in diseases account for some different outcomes in women and men? For example, recent research reveals that cardiovascular disease manifests differently in women, making it difficult to detect with diagnostic tests developed for men. We know that there are differences in the incidence of certain diseases that are determined by gender roles; for example, WHO found differences in tropical diseases when it (belatedly, in the 1990s) studied women separately from men. But are diseases also determined by biological differences between the sexes? This question is analogous to the one being asked about the need for research on the diseases and treatment of African Americans; despite conclusive evidenced that race is a social construct, not a biological reality, some researchers believe that there are race-based biological differences in disease.[6]

Would biological differences matter or do discriminatory beliefs and practices override biology? Feminists start from the premise that disease is a natural, biological reality that is socially produced and socially defined; both global and local economic environments influence disease (Sundari Ravindran 1997b). Yet in South Asia, the perception that women are of no economic utility underlies gender-based health differences. Fikree and Pasha (2004) claim that gender—based on social, cultural, and, in some cases, legal constructs and practices—overrides the biological advantage of being born female. Education and improved economic circumstances alone are unlikely to change practices that have become culturally, socially and, in some cases, legally enshrined.

Another question is: does the sex or gender of the person who designs research projects matter? Would more funding of research projects designed by women and lesbians change the design and targets of projects and affect the findings and outcomes? Are the research priorities of women and men different? This question is analogous to the one gays asked (and answered in the affirmative) when AIDS first appeared in their community. Feminists claim that the core of feminist methodology lies in its recognition of the power relations inherent in the research process and its attempt to make these relations transparent. Male researchers rarely reflect on issues of difference between the researcher and the subjects of research or allow the people being studied to determine the research agenda and process ensuring that the research topic concerns them (Klugman 1994).

A third set of questions: does research on women's health require a different methodology from research on men's health? The crude measures of socioeconomic status and other socially structured determinants of health currently in use fail to capture differences in gendered social conditions affecting health. They ignore the impact of cumulative psychosocial adversity and are blind to structural economic reforms that pose additional socially based, gender-specific risks to health (Astbury 2002).

Cross-sectional research is not as effective as longitudinal research in understanding how changes in household social conditions mediate the course of illness and whether it becomes chronic.[7] Qualitative methodology overcomes some of these issues and avoids the objectification of women, which is a common fault in traditional, biomedical methodologies. In another context, that of biological experimentation, Lewontin (2000) finds that methodology determines the kinds of questions that biologists ask as well as the explanations they offer; methodological limitations of experiments are confused with the correct explanations of the phenomenon. One wonders whether the same sort of limitations have operated in research on women's health.

In health as in other fields, feminist research asks new questions and seeks new answers about women's perceptions and experiences (Oakley and Mitchell 1976). Some examples are the Women's Health Project in South Africa, which conducted research on how women feel about contraception and contraceptive services as a contribution to wider discussions on health policy (Women's Health Project Newsletter 1992); the Women's Health Research Network has focused on infertility in Nigeria, a condition that many women experience and many more fear, in an effort to develop more effective public policies to control sexually transmitted diseases (Kisseka 1990); and the International Women's Health Coalition, which has commissioned experts to conduct literature reviews on reproductive tract infections in women (Germain et al. 1992). At the conceptual level, researchers formed the International Reproductive Rights Action Group in 1992 to conduct research on the meaning of "reproductive rights" to women in Brazil, Egypt, Mexico, Malaysia, Nigeria, the Philippines, and the United States (Petchesky and Judd 1998).

Research Ethics

An additional question arises because of ingrained discrimination against women and the way industries have coopted our activism (for example, around infertility): do the ethical standards applied to research differ for studies on women and men? And, following from that question, do different ethical standards govern the use of research results when treating women and men? Studies of research ethics often focus narrowly on protocols and do not call into question larger issues of inequitable global relations, the structure of markets, and the sources of funding, even though these factors are often determinant (Benatar and Singer 2000). Historical perspective is also often lacking, especially a perspective on the role medicine has played in generating racialized narratives of global citizenship (Craddock 2004). Good and ethical research protocols may still leave intact the status quo: unequal distribution of medical resources, unequal distribution of disease, and unequal power in tackling these issues.

Research protocols involving women in the global South have often violated the Declaration of Helsinki, the ethical guidelines that govern international research.[8] The Declaration of Helsinki demands informed participation of volunteers, the reasonable likelihood that the people studied stand to benefit from the research, and equal standards of medical care during research (in technical terms, the testing of new methods against the best current prophylactic, diagnostic, and therapeutic methods). The World Medical Association underscores this last point: researchers should not use placebos in clinical trials when drugs proven to treat or cure the condition under study already exist.[9]

Puerto Rican women were among the first human guinea pigs enlisted in the clinical trials of the contraceptive pill in the 1950s, before the adoption of the Declaration of Helsinki in 1964, but after widespread acceptance of the 1948 Nuremberg Code on medical experimentation. Adopted during the Nuremberg military trials of Nazi war criminals, the code established the absolute requirement of voluntary consent including an understanding of potential hazards to health (www.nihtraining.com/ohsrsite/info/sheet11.html accessed 20 March 2007).

In Puerto Rico, researchers pressed hundreds of mostly poor and uneducated women to take the pill experimentally, not knowing what the health consequences might be. When female medical students at the University of San Juan refused to assist in the project, their teachers punished them by lowering their grades (Seaman 1995).[10] By 1960, researchers were conducting clinical trials in Haiti, Mexico, Hong Kong, and Sri Lanka. The exploitation of women in the South who have participated in clinical drug trials raises larger questions of social justice and human rights. One question is whether medical associations, which do not have the power to enforce existing guidelines, can address these larger issues by rewriting ethical guidelines for research practice, or whether we need more comprehensive changes in the status quo of global economic and political practice to address these questions (Craddock 2004).

The few studies that examine the conduct of research ethics committees suggest that, wary of socially sensitive research and studies of abuses of institutional power, ethics committees tend to reject such proposals. Apartheid provided the ideological framework for decades of South African health research that allowed racism, sexism, and heterosexism to masquerade as "scientific objectivity." With the democratic transition, de Gruchy and Lewin (2001) tried to obtain approval of research into how health professionals treated lesbians and gay men in the South African military during the apartheid era.

> The [ethics] committee questioned the "scientific validity" of the study, viewing it as having a "political" rather than a "scientific" purpose. They objected to the framing of the research topic within a human rights discourse and appeared to be concerned that the research might lead to action against health professionals who committed human rights abuses against lesbians and gay men during apartheid. (de Gruchy and Lewin 2001, 865)

One women's group focuses specifically on these issues. Feminist Approaches to Bioethics (FAB) is an international network devoted to developing a more inclusive theory of bioethics encompassing the standpoints and experiences of women and other marginalized social groups, to examining presuppositions embedded in the dominant bioethical discourse that privilege those already empowered, and to creating new methodologies and strategies responsive to the disparate conditions of women's lives across the globe (www.msu.edu/nhlinde/fab). They held their 2006 conference, Gender Justice and Women's Rights in Healthcare, in Beijing in conjunction with the 8th World Congress of Bioethics, at which they organized a joint plenary and concurrent sessions with the International Association of Bioethics (IAB).

Two Research Cultures: Arts and Sciences

The attempt to answer the question why medical research so often ignores women begins from the premise that social status determines women's health to a greater extent than men's health, and that, in general, women's lower social and economic status causes women to experience more health problems and to have less access to treatment for them.

The second premise is that the culture of the humanities—including the arts and the social sciences—is fundamentally separate from the culture of physical sciences (as C.P. Snow famously described in a 1959 lecture). Researchers may receive education in both arts and sciences but rarely across these disciplines in a multidisciplinary approach to problem solving or problem-based learning. Researchers from the liberal arts and medical sciences rarely train together in teams and therefore have little opportunity to learn constructive collaboration. As a result, scientifically trained medical personnel rarely understand social scientists, and the distrust is mutual.

The educational experience offers few opportunities to build a common vocabulary and mutual respect for each other's skills. Social scientists often try to mimic physics—the paradigm for science—while people with lab training have a bias against the social scientists they perceive as less than precise. Lab workers do not understand that social scientists cannot ethically experiment on human communities as lab scientists can on animals, or that it is impossible to control inputs and outputs in human communities or even know what all the influential factors are. Physical scientists hold a bias against qualitative research. In social science, a hierarchy of values places the most quantitative field—economics—at the top and the most qualitative fields like cultural anthropology or women's studies at the bottom.

The consequences of this binary split for health are serious indeed. If hard scientists, practicing medical doctors, and social scientists had come together at the beginning of the AIDS epidemic, for example, they might have explored and understood the public health implications of urban redevelopment, public housing, and municipal policies described in the case of the South Bronx (see chapter 3). Reasons for the binary split go back to the origins of public health and social science. Historically, public health was a branch of medicine, and schools of public health required a prior degree in medicine for admission; only later did the schools accept a nursing degree, and only in the United States. Yet public health personnel are most in need of the principles of social science. Public health workers must understand nonmedical aspects of health—health economics, sociology, political organization, policy—and they need to understand community dynamics of racism, sexism, and class prejudice so critical to successful public health work. Public health workers also need to be aware that they wield the police powers of the state and that their knowledge of communities can be used against as well as for communities, especially if workers accept victim-blaming analyses of problems.

Without social science training that goes beyond behavioral science to change people's habits, we will continue to see a narrow concentration on biological causes of disease, and we will see research projects that study one disease at a time, ignoring synergies and clusters. Extensive discrimination against women (whether intentional or unwitting) will also continue. The biases outlined here are cumulative; they most affect communities at the bottom of the economic ladder and at the bottom of gender, racial, and ethnic hierarchies. These are precisely the groups most in need of public health and public protection.

CHAPTER FIVE

The Sexual Politics of Violence against Women

Sexuality

Sexuality is at the center of women's health. Sexuality affects reproduction, women's mental health, social identity, and general well-being. To the patriarchal mind, sexuality evokes danger, disease, and death: the risks of overpopulation, sexually transmitted diseases, and sexual violence. Control of women's sexuality is critical to reproduction of the labor force (the production and socialization of the next generation), including the armed forces. Society undertakes to control women's sexuality in part to control women's productive labor, both paid and unpaid. Rigid gender roles are an expression of this effort to control men's and women's sexuality: they dictate how women and men express their sexuality, what work each gender must do, what work either may do, and what work either may not do. Society uses its control of women's sexuality to perpetuate the social order, for example by specifying that women bear children and also rear and socialize them in the customs of their culture.

Sexuality is not just sexual activity; it is also an identity. Sexuality lies at the intersection of sex and gender, of the biological and the cultural construction of womanhood and manhood. Power relations among racial and ethnic groups, classes and castes, religious and age groups are among the factors that affect men and women's sexuality. These factors are at the base of gender relations, which are relations of power between women and men, between older and younger women, and among men.

We need to break down the concepts of social control of sexuality and social construction of gender into the components of society so that we can understand the meaning of women's subordination in its cultural context. Society comprises, at a minimum, the state and the family. For women in the global South, for women in conquered communities of indigenous people, and for the descendants of slaves, the state contains the colonial legacy as well as earlier state functions embedded in customary law and later revisions made by the postcolonial state. This complex legacy encodes the task of the colonial state to articulate and preserve those codes of conduct that Western systems of knowledge had characterized as colonial peoples' signs of "otherness." The state articulated these codes of honor and shame, purity and pollution, and hierarchy through anthropological and administrative knowledge and state practices (Das 1995). In the process, the state invested these codes with new authority and made them much more rigid.

Distinctive religious or ethical codes dominate family systems everywhere. Three regimes—patriarchy, marriage, and fertility—characterize these diverse arrangements (Therborn 2004). Patriarchy is dominant in family systems, which command the rules of marriage, regulate sexual relations, and set the norms of reproduction. A regime that invests family power in fathers and husbands, patriarchy is a universal pattern in retreat. Over the course of the twentieth century, patriarchy yielded to the upheavals of two world wars, revolutions in Russia and China, and the worldwide student revolts of the 1960s (with practice usually trailing behind policy). Virtually universal marriage continues with two significant exceptions—Western Europe and those parts of Latin America that had mines and plantations in the colonial era where formal unions were few and out-of-wedlock births numerous. The main changes are the rising age of first marriage and higher divorce rates. Fertility has undergone the greatest change, dramatically falling in Europe and North America between the 1880s and 1930s (in the absence of state policy and contraceptive technology) and abruptly dropping in Latin America, Asia, and Africa from the mid-1970s (under the pressure of state policy and the widespread availability of contraceptive technology). It follows that "the astonishing fall in birthrates in most of the underdeveloped world has been the product of a historic collapse in patriarchal authority, as its powers of life and death have been transferred to the state, which now determines how many are born and how many survive" (Anderson 2005, 30).

In nations that had a strong state before colonialists seized power, the interaction of the family and the state was a constant preoccupation of regulators and religious authorities. Women's sexuality was always a target, one element of maintaining state control. In nineteenth-century

Egypt the modern state (beginning with Muhammad 'Ali, 1805–1848) introduced educational and health policies that ostensibly benefited and liberated women (Hatem 2000). At the same time, the state was establishing its right and ability to control women's reproductive capacity, to determine the uses of women's reproductive skills, and ultimately to deny women autonomy—all in the service of pronatalist policies (Hatem 2000). This project was not without Western influences as the Egyptian government recruited European doctors.

Society controls women's sexuality (more or less tightly, everywhere) through ideology, law, family values, and the sexual division of labor. Social sanctions—dress codes, cosmetics, the hours at which one may appear in public, the public places one may appear (unaccompanied), one's comportment and demeanor at all times and places, and gossip— operate to keep women "in line." Many other customs illustrate the same point: restrictions on women's and girls' education, training, and occupation; rituals of puberty, menstruation, and childbirth; religious teachings (about birth control and contraception, for example), which may reinforce or conflict with the dominant culture; heterosexist dominance within the family, school, community, and workplace; and universal expectations of marriage, motherhood, and (in most societies) monogamy.

Societies also regulate access to knowledge about sexuality and bodily functions, informally by silencing discussion and formally by restricting sex education in the schools or by interfering with the work of non-governmental organizations like the International Planned Parenthood Federation. As a result, secrecy surrounds human sexuality, especially female sexuality, contributing to violence against women. In Rajasthan, India, the state-run Women's Development Programme sponsored a health project in the late 1980s (Sawhney 1999). The chosen themes were fertility, sexuality, and childbirth. After six months the medical establishment and higher government authorities expressed their disapproval, accusing the project of instigating and corrupting rural women, of failing to motivate them to accept family planning, and therefore of working against national interests. Doctors did not approve of women controlling their fertility through increased awareness of fertility cycles; they wanted them to accept the contraceptive methods that the state promoted.

Social and legal sanctions link sexuality to sexism and sustain discrimination against women. The differential enrollment and treatment of girls and boys in schools and of women and men in health care facilities and in employment institutionalize sexism. The use of force, threats of force, and legal controls of women's sexuality support social sanctions on women's deviance from engrained norms. Sexual harassment, domestic violence, and how police, the courts, and hospital systems respond to violence against women are all examples of sanctions.

Some people believe that gender violence is inevitable, but all over the world women are organizing against it. Women in almost every country have united against society's attempts to control their sexuality with violence (Schuler 1992). Women have mobilized against sexual violence and rape, confronting men who batter, reclaiming spaces of exclusion, and demonstrating publicly in mass rallies. They have created strategies for reform of laws, practices, and attitudes regarding violence against women; and they have already accomplished much, changing legislation and shifting men's attitudes.

The Asia-Pacific Resource and Research Center for Women (ARROW) reviewed the record of seven Southeast Asian countries and found that women's nongovernmental organizations have done the most advocacy work on the issue of violence against women. "This is the area where most progress has been made by government—both in the revision or development of new laws to protect women (from sexual harassment, domestic violence, rape) and to punish offenders, as well as providing government health services to women survivors" (Abdullah 2003, 34). Despite this encouraging survey, Amnesty International, in its 2005 annual assessment of human rights, reported abuses against women from almost every country in Asia and noted a long list of places in which women's rights had deteriorated. UNIFEM (the UN Development Fund for Women) reported that violence against women in South Asia was on the rise, based on cases reported to the police (Bhalla 2005).

Violence against Women

Violence against women takes many forms—social, economic, political, and cultural; all forms effectively restrict women's liberty. Unpacking the categories of violence and considering each one separately permits us to explore the extent and heterogeneity of this pervasive aggression. Women most commonly report acts of social and interpersonal violence; these include domestic violence, rape (by spouses, partners, dates, or acquaintances as well as by strangers), psychological and emotional abuse, sexual harassment, use of sexist language, stalking, incest, child abuse, child pornography, and child prostitution. Most of the literature on violence against women deals with social and interpersonal violence.

Women's groups are analyzing and organizing against economic and systemic violence. Often related to domestic violence, economic violence deprives women of independence and can determine women's options and their ability to leave an abusive relationship. Economic violence includes laws that limit women's property rights as well as their autonomy in matters of business and banking; it also encompasses discrimination against women in the labor force—unequal pay, the glass ceiling, restrictions on types of work and work hours, and denial of paid leave to accommodate maternity and maternal obligations. The broader category of systemic violence covers the violence of slavery, which is the theft of women's productive and reproductive labor; the violence of racial segregation and apartheid; the violence of colonialism; and the structural violence of poverty, unemployment, and homelessness.

Women added political violence to the debates on violence against women as they considered the meaning of citizenship. Examples of political violence are: the denial of full citizenship to women; women's lack of political representation (enabling male-dominated legislatures to pass laws inimical to the interests of women); the wrongful imprisonment, detention, and enslavement of women; their forced eviction from their homes and homelands; and their statelessness.

Discussions of the universality of human rights as defined by the United Nations have created a fourth category, cultural violence. Figuring in the debates are customs that deny women's individual identity, separate from their father's or husband's, and ignore women's multiple roles, which some would call identities, or impose an alien identity, as when women are absorbed into a husband's family/clan/religion/nationality; as well, activists are examining the practice of making women the symbol of a culture. Arguments continue about whether customs judged harmful to women's health by today's standards are cultural rites to which women have a right or constitute violence against women's bodily integrity.

All forms of violence—social, economic, political, and cultural—affect women's health directly and indirectly. The list of health consequences from domestic violence alone is extensive: physical injury, depression, suicide, gynecological problems, and complications of pregnancy (especially when men direct violence against women during pregnancy) including vaginal bleeding, premature labor, low birth weight, miscarriage, and stillbirth (Garcia-Moreno et al. 2003). A survey of Australian women revealed that 36 percent have experienced violence in a relationship and that domestic violence was the leading cause of premature death and ill health in women aged 15 to 44 (Amnesty International 2005). Death or severe injuries claim hundreds of Afghan women who have set fire to themselves to escape violence in the home or forced marriage; some women cut their wrists, others swallow poison or hang themselves (Gall 2004). Many in the health community still think these are individual medical problems rather than public health issues, and that public health workers can do little about the health consequences of gender violence.

Social and Interpersonal Violence

Acts of social and interpersonal violence occur in public as well as domestic settings; acts in public settings include street rapes and teacher-pupil abuse (consideration of institutional abuse appears in the section on political violence). Of interest here is how discussions of gender-based violence often narrow to immediate concerns of social and interpersonal violence. This contraction occurs because interpersonal violence is so widespread that women everywhere identify with it, and because other forms of violence—economic, political, and cultural—are much harder to analyze.

Some people think that domestic violence is not a women's but a men's issue, as this example suggests. A Mauritian nongovernmental organization, S.O.S. Femmes, has carried out a wide range of activities since 1990 to raise public awareness about gender-based violence and build a culture of zero-tolerance. After considering the primary causes of violence and analyzing the unequal relationships between men and women, S.O.S. Femmes decided to engage in dialogue with men on women's rights, sexism, and the gender division of such tasks as bringing up children and caring for the sick and elderly (Gungaloo 2003). Their analysis shows that the basis of violence against women is economic and political norms, social and cultural customs, and religious attitudes. Mauritian men believe that women are inferior and should be submissive, in particular that they should submit to men's will. To challenge prevalent notions of masculinity and femininity, S.O.S. Femmes decided to invite men to redefine masculinity, to revisit their traditionally ascribed roles and duties, and to recognize that they still hold and wield power at all levels. If men and women want to build just and nonviolent societies and families, they need to overturn and transform these power relationships. Women cannot simply ask men to prevent gender-based violence and to protect "their" women because this is not about good men and bad men. Gender-based violence is a structural problem having its roots in the gendered social construction of society.

Domestic Violence

Many patriarchal societies do not perceive domestic violence as an issue, and they accuse the women who raise it of attempting to break up families. Victims of domestic violence seldom receive support or help from family members who blame them and hold them responsible for the violence. Religious authorities, police, the courts, and the medical profession are likely to echo or amplify this rejection, leaving women nowhere to go but back home to their abusers. Paradoxically, people who observe battered women remaining in abusive relationships often wonder aloud, "Why don't they just leave?"

Domestic violence appears to be so common around the world that women's groups in almost every country are addressing it. Some work through legislative channels, as does Vimochana, an Indian women's organization in Bangalore that pushes for new laws to combat domestic violence. Others work in the institutions that are supposed to treat or protect battered women such as the health services (especially mental health institutions), police and courts (like the Advice Desk located at the University of Natal Westville campus in Durban, South Africa). Still others provide direct services such as shelters for battered women (like Friends of Women in Thailand, which first opened a shelter in 1985).

India still lacks comprehensive legislation on domestic violence, according to Amnesty International (2005). Indian women in groups like Majilis, a women's legal rights charity, have lobbied and staged street demonstrations for the past ten years to persuade the government to recognize that the cruelty of husbands may be criminal. Indian women's groups claim that one in three women face some form of domestic violence, yet most remain silent; 50,703 cases were reported in 2003 but the real figure could be ten times higher (Bhalla 2005).

Beyond the widely publicized phenomenon of "dowry deaths"—the burning of brides whose families gave less gold, cash, and consumer goods than were demanded as part of marriage arrangements—Indian women have found the need to look at the more generalized and common practice of wife-beating and abuse by husbands and in-laws. In March 2002, the Government of India introduced the Prevention from Domestic Violence Bill, which had many prejudicial requirements such as counseling for women who complain of domestic violence. The bill failed to recognize complaints of a single attack as an instance of domestic violence (the battery must be habitual), and it failed to provide any remedy for victims of domestic violence. Finally, it granted men immunity if they beat their wife to protect themselves, their property, or the property of another person. Confronting this backward step, the Lawyers Collective of the Women's Rights Initiative, after extensive nation-wide consultations, drafted a bill, which the Indian government largely rejected.

In 2005, the Indian Parliament considered a new bill focusing not on penalizing the offender but on protecting and compensating the victim by awarding a share of the abuser's property and salary as well as damages for physical abuse, medical and legal costs. The bill redefines domestic violence to include physical, sexual, verbal, emotional, and economic abuse and makes it easier for victims to complain and police and the judiciary to take action. It also mandates the appointment of protection officers and private service providers to help abused women get medical and legal aid and a safe place to stay. The issue of women's rights to residence is crucial in cases where a woman's courage to lodge a complaint with the police leaves her homeless. The law will protect the rights of victims to secure a house or live in her married home (Bhalla 2005).

If fire by kerosene stoves is the weapon frequently used against women in Indian domestic disputes, the weapon of choice in Bangladesh is sulfuric acid, used not to kill but to disfigure women. From March 1998 to March 1999, the police recorded 174 acid attacks (Bearak 2000). Nariphokko, a women's rights group, has kept statistics: 80 attacks in 1996, 117 in 1997, 130 in 1998, and 153 between January and October 2004. The police rarely arrest attackers and the courts never try most of those arrested. Although the maximum penalty is death, the state has never executed anyone. Some Bangladeshi villagers resort to customary law, convening a *shaleesh* or informal court of village elders to mediate between the parties and reach agreement on a cash settlement in compensation. The trope of the disappointed lover who takes revenge on his self-selected bride masks the reality of unresolved property disputes between families in which young women are vulnerable targets (Zafrin Chowdhury personal communication, 2 May 2005).

Violence in Immigrant Communities

Domestic violence festers in immigrant communities at the intersection of gender and ethnicity. Immigration places stress on relationships because it changes gender roles; women who work outside the home, earning money and learning different relationship styles, may find a new independence from which to challenge their men. Others arriving from countries where women are subordinate to men may be isolated, alone, and easily victimized. In arranged marriages, brides do not meet their husbands before the wedding, and with their natal family far away they may have no one to whom they can appeal. Abusers often use isolation as a tactic to cut women off from sympathetic networks, making women in immigrant communities especially vulnerable. Immigrant women rarely know more than the language of their birth, compounding the difficulty of finding services. They may have no knowledge of the country in which they are living. Where a wife's status is dependent on her husband's immigration status, the dangers of domestic violence intensify because any attempt at escape from an abusive situation puts the woman in a legal limbo. In the United States, for example, the law requires women who come to the country through husbands who are U.S. citizens to hold "conditional" status for two years, preventing many immigrant women from seeking redress (Coomaraswamy 2001).

Samira Bellil (2002), an Algerian immigrant who wrote about being gang raped when she was 14-years-old, brought to light violence against women and girls in immigrant communities in France.[1] She had fallen in love when she was 14-years-old and agreed to have sex with her boyfriend; immediately afterward he passed her on to his waiting friends who beat and gang raped her throughout the night. A month later, the most violent rapist, K, dragged her off a train by her hair, while other passengers looked the other way, and she was gang-raped again. Still she said nothing until three friends said K had attacked them too. Bellil learned that her experience was far from unique; passing around a girlfriend was as banal as passing around a joint. The shame of a gang rape is crippling: most girls do not dare speak for fear of reprisals like apartments burned down and threats to younger sisters. Bellil reported the rapes, joining a tiny minority of women who do so. She did not know that she could prosecute the men for raping, sodomizing, and forcing her to fellate three boys; she did not know these were crimes punishable by French law (George 2004). The court sentenced K to eight years in prison for rape. Bellil says that women are the guardians of honor in the deprived housing projects on the outskirts of French cities populated by immigrants. Girls have to be virgins; they have to study at home, look after the men, and never go out. Doing anything else makes one a slut. "If you want a 'French' life, if you want to go out, wear make-up, you get a reputation" (quoted in George 2003).

In February 2003, women from all over France found their voice, rallying for a five-week march through more than 20 French cities with the war cry *Ni Putes Ni Soumises* (Neither Prostitutes Nor Doormats). The march began, symbolically, in Vitry-sur-Seine, where a gang of boys set 17-year-old Sohane Benziane alight with lighter fuel, burning her to death. The march made more than 20 stops all over the country and ended in Paris on March 8th, International Women's Day, where it attracted a crowd of 20,000. Fadela Amara, director of the grassroots organization House of Friends (*La Maison des Potes*), has been working in housing projects on the city outskirts (*banlieues*) for two decades. "The public has no idea what's been happening. When they talk about the *banlieue*, they talk about crime. They never talk about women. All the rights feminism won stop at the gates of the *banlieue*" (quoted in George 2003).

Domestic violence in immigrant communities accounts for many of the murders of women. Intimate partners are more likely to kill a woman in New York City than a stranger, especially if she is young and foreign-born, according to a New York City Health Department report, "Femicide in New York City 1995–2002," which analyzes 339 such deaths (Bernstein and Kaufman 2004). Lovers and husbands were responsible for almost 60 percent of the deaths of women between 20 and 50 years old, and such victims were 87 percent more likely than those killed by strangers to be foreign-born. Nearly 60 percent were killed in their own homes. The report documents the vulnerability of immigrant women in a number of ways: intimate partners killed 57 percent of all foreign-born victims, and just over 50 percent of all the women killed by intimate partners were immigrants; but immigrant women were only 35 percent of those killed by others.

The message has gotten out to groups that work with immigrant women. South Asian women in the United States have organized groups in many of the major centers of Asian immigration like California and New Jersey as well as cities like New York, Chicago, Washington, Philadelphia, and Austin; the groups pressure the U.S. government to pass protective legislation and offer services to abused women from their communities (Abraham 2000). Manavi, based in New Jersey, was the first South Asian women's organization to address the issue of domestic violence in the mid-1980s. Sakhi (meaning female friend in Hindi) is a support group based in New York City run by South Asian women to help women from India, Bangladesh, Pakistan, Nepal, and Indian communities from the Caribbean. Founded in 1990, Sakhi teaches women about their rights and how to exercise them in the United States; it offers such services as finding a place to live, language assistance, legal advice in court cases, and liaison with New York City services.

Violence in Subordinate Communities

States and social structures institutionalize discrimination based on nationality, ethnicity, race, religion, and language, decreasing the rights and remedies available to women and increasing women's vulnerability to violence and abuse. The United Nations refers to the experience of discrimination on more than one ground as intersectionality, the idea that racism, patriarchy, economic disadvantage, and other discriminatory systems create layers of inequality that structure the relative positions of women and men, racial and other groups. Intersectionality describes the way that specific acts and policies create burdens that flow along these intersecting axes, creating a dynamic of disempowerment (Coomaraswamy 2001).

The UN distinguishes three types of intersectional subordination: targeted discrimination (ethnically motivated gender-specific forms of violence; rape in civil conflicts is an example); compound discrimination (discrimination against women who are also members of a subordinate racial or ethnic group); and structural discrimination (where policies intersect with underlying structures of inequality to create a compound burden for particularly vulnerable women). An example of structural discrimination is the experience of battered Asian women who seek protection and redress from the criminal justice system in England but find they are aiding the state in implementing racist immigration policies; deportation orders against their men put the women in the position of legitimizing institutional racism (Coomaraswamy 2001). Structural discrimination also puts pressure on indigenous women or women from racially or ethnically marginalized groups not to report violence for fear of greater group stigmatization.

Women of color, members of racial and national minorities in the United States, are more vulnerable to abuse from institutions as well as partners than are white women (Ritchie 1996). Stereotypes about women of color contribute to this abuse. Racial, ethnic, and class differences are manifest in each form of violence against women, as are age, ableness, and sexuality. The individual focus of research, policy, and service on domestic violence misses the interplay between individual and institutional racism and domestic violence. Like Asian women in England, battered women of color in the United States who seek protection from the police face a dilemma in a racist society in which police use coercive and violent means of criminal enforcement.

Honor Killings

When the concepts of honor and shame attach to women's bodies, they suggest the pervasive archaism of moral values. Codes of conduct from earlier periods of social organization distinguish societies that follow them from other cultures, especially in the industrial world. In the discourses on honor and shame and on personal and family behavioral codes, the role of European powers in inscribing these values during the colonial era becomes invisible; colonial authorities presented the codes as archaic and immutable. In ethnographic studies the role of the state in enforcing such codes disappears; in the foreground ethnographers place village cultures, removed from the modern world. I want to emphasize how much of what commentators write about women in the global South reduces complex historical interactions between colonial powers and conquered societies to harmful customs that oppress women. These customs then become emblematic, and when journalists write about honor killings or rape in the global South, they incriminate entire societies (see Fisher 2002). In the North reporters individualize the same crimes and refer to them as crimes of passion (see Lyall 2002). Honor killings remain coded as cultural violence, as if they were categorically different from other forms of domestic violence.

Radhika Coomaraswamy (2001, 4), Special Rapporteur of the UN Commission on Human Rights on violence against women, makes an additional point about women who challenge "traditions" that violate women's rights from within communities:

> Community members may invoke customary and religious prac-
> tices to justify violence directed towards women. This has impor-
> tant gender and race implications because such justifications tend to
> (mis)appropriate arguments regarding Western cultural imperial-
> ism. Those seeking to justify gender-related violence may accuse
> challengers of imposing Western cultural norms upon their own
> distinct cultures. For example, opposition to so-called "honour
> killings" in Jordan or to female circumcision in parts of Africa and
> the African diaspora are characterized as being led by "Western"
> feminists. In addition to minimizing [the importance of] violence
> against women, such appeals to the communities' shared racial,
> national, cultural or religious identity can serve to rationalize non-
> interference by the State.

Every year men murder women and girls in the name of family honor, and they cloak the deaths with the legitimacy of "tradition" to escape condemnation for their brutality. In Mediterranean societies, the Arab world, and the Balkans, men can justify their crimes with claims that these women are misusing their sexuality and causing the family to suf-fer shame and disgrace. In fact, the women's behavior may be anything from attending school to running away from home, breaches of gender roles but not necessarily sexual transgressions. The common thread in the range of women's unacceptable acts—from defying dress codes to engaging in premarital sex—is the inability of these women to marry once gossip has ruined their reputations. At least one observer believes the persistence of honor crimes to be a consequence of the modern desegregation of gendered social spaces, rendering the concept of sexual honor ambiguous (Abu-Odeh 2000). But when a 25-year-old man rapes a 4-year-old girl and her family leaves her to bleed to death because they believe she has dishonored them (Ruggi 2000), it is hard to credit explanations that accuse women of transgressive behavior. In the binary world of honor and shame, women have shame, men have honor.

Men's ability to justify their criminal behavior and escape punishment is encoded in law, not just custom. The Turkish penal code mandates a 24 year prison term for premeditated murder, but "severe provocation" reduces the term to 15 years in honor killings, and the young age of the murderer can reduce it even further, leading some families to assign this task to teenage boys (Düzkan and Koçali 2000).[2] Official records show that 43 women were victims of honor killings in 2004, but human rights activists say the number is far greater: families tend to report deaths as suicides or they file missing persons reports (Arsu 2005). In Turkey many women's groups—Equality-Watch Committee, the Purple Roof (Women's Shelter Foundation), the Gaziantep Women's Platform, and the Association to Support Contemporary Living—are leading the combat against custom and law, sending their members to attend courtroom trials to defend murdered women. A new penal code ratified in September 2004 eliminated "protection of family honor" as a mitigating circumstance in murder trials and introduced heavier penalties for honor killing convictions, but "unjust provocation" is still available as a defense that could be invoked (Arsu 2005).

The 1960 Jordanian penal code exempts a man who murders his wife caught in an act of adultery because the court judges his act one of self-defense—he has defended his life, his honor, or someone else's honor (Ruggi 2000). The court may also reduce the penalty for a man who murders one of his female ascendants or descendants or sisters caught in an "unlawful bed" (Abu-Odeh 2000).

The Albadeel Coalition, formed in 1994, works to end violence against women in the Palestinian community in Israel; it publicly debates this taboo subject, calling for indictment and punishment of killers and honoring the memory of the dead women.[3] The Palestinian case is especially poignant because it raises the question how a society can interrogate itself and hold open debates on reform in the midst of a war and under intense pressure from external powers. It seems to me that women are more open to change in times of war because circumstances have already forced them into unaccustomed activities that question traditional gender roles, but men may be more resistant to change because war challenges their masculinity.

In this passage from her novel, *Regeneration*, about the First World War, Pat Barker vividly describes the challenges to masculinity.

> One of the paradoxes of the war—one of the many—was that this most brutal of conflicts should set up a relationship between officers and men that was . . . domestic. Caring . . . maternal. And that wasn't the only trick the war had played. Mobilization. The Great Adventure. They'd been *mobilized* into holes in the ground so constricted they could hardly move. And the Great Adventure—the real life equivalent of all the adventure stories they'd devoured as boys—consisted of crouching in a dugout, waiting to be killed. The war that had promised so much in the way of "manly" activity had actually delivered "feminine" passivity, and on a scale that their mothers and sisters had scarcely known. No wonder they broke down. (Barker 1991, 107)

Rape

Debates about rape center on whether it is an act of individual deviance or an extension of other learned and accepted male behaviors. For some women, rape statistics speak volumes about the low value of women: surveys show that 14 to 20 percent of women in Canada, Korea, New Zealand, and the United States will experience a completed rape during their lifetime (PANOS 1998). Evidence that rape is widely condoned suggests that in some cases it is a violent method for keeping women in their place, a product of patriarchal society. Often, a rape victim's body language and the way she dresses directly affect the opinion of police, prosecutors, judges, and jurors, even though data on the rape of babies and elderly women bear out the irrelevance of such criteria to whether a female becomes a victim of a gender crime and whether she is credible. More than half of all rapes in the United States occur to victims under 18 years of age and over one-fourth before the victim is 11-years-old. Women over 65 are also victims.

As with other acts of social and interpersonal violence, rape can occur in public as well as private settings. Men commit "public rapes" while serving in their official capacity in prisons, in war zones, and in refugee camps (the last two are discussed in the sections on wartime violence and refugees). The experience of rape is socially constructed; that is, how society reacts, what the police response is, how the courts handle the case, whether the woman is blamed or the man is prosecuted, whether medical care is readily available from concerned specialists, and whether the morning-after pill, HIV testing, and abortion are available partly determine how women experience rape. Sympathetic treatment and better services lessen the trauma of the experience.

When officials order rape as punishment, it is "public rape." In Meerwala Jatoi, Pakistan, a village council decreed the gang rape of Mukhtaran Bibi, a poor, low-caste, 28-year-old, illiterate, divorced woman, to avenge a crime allegedly committed by her 12-year-old brother (Fisher 2002). This was a double crime against the woman as it punished her for someone else's alleged act and decreed cruel and unusual punishment. According to Beena Sarwar (2002), a Pakistani journalist, the government of Pakistan "routinely turns a blind eye" to justice rendered by such councils, called *panchayat* or *jirga*; so the council members "were certain they could get away with it, of course." The government does not support its own police chiefs and district commissioners who attempt to end these judgments, which decide so-called "private" matters of land and family disputes. After the rape by four high-caste men, council members forced Bibi to walk home naked while some 300 villagers watched. A local imam, Abdul Razzaq, revealed the incident when he condemned it during Friday prayers; journalists then publicized it, forcing the national government to arrest the alleged rapists and members of the tribal council.

President Pervez Musharraf presented Ms. Mukhtaran with the equivalent of $8,300. Bibi, who had never gone to school herself, used the money to build two village schools, one for girls and another for boys, because, she said, education is the best way to achieve social change. The girls' school is named for her, and in 2004 she studied in its fourth-grade class. "Why should I have spent the money on myself?" she asked, adding, "This way the money is helping all the girls, all the children" (Rizvi 2004). Unfortunately that is not the end of the story.

In March 2005, Pakistan's Supreme Court, its highest court, agreed to decide the case of the six men sentenced to death, after the High Court in Lahore had overturned the convictions of five of the men and reduced the sixth to life in prison. The High Court ruled on March 3rd and on March 4th the Federal Shariah Court, the nation's highest Islamic tribunal, threw out the acquittal and reinstated the death sentences, a ruling the Supreme Court deemed unconstitutional (*New York Times*

15 March 2005). Within ten days, a local judge released four of the five acquitted men (*New York Times* 16 March 2005); then the police re-arrested the four men (*New York Times* 19 March 2005); and three months later a Lahore High Court panel ordered the release of 12 men behind bars (*New York Times* 11 June 2005). At the same time, the government placed Mukhtaran Bibi under house arrest, confiscated the passport for which she had applied, and stopped her from leaving the country (*The Guardian Unlimited* 14 June 2005). Amnesty International had invited Bibi to speak in England and the United States, but President Musharraf was afraid she might tarnish the image of Pakistan. He told the Auckland Foreign Correspondents' Club that nongovernmental organizations are "Westernised fringe elements" that "are as bad as the Islamic extremists" (*Off Road Pakistan* 18 June 2005). Under pressure from the U.S. government, the Pakistani government lifted its travel restrictions (*New York Times* 16 June 2005). On 20 July 2005, Bibi was still on the exit control list, prohibiting her departure, and still not in possession of her passport, which authorities continued to hold. Then in August 2005, the Pakistani government awarded Mukhtaran Bibi the Fatima Jinnah gold medal for bravery and courage, and in November *Glamour* magazine named her their Woman of the Year. In January 2006, she published her memoir in French[4] and traveled to France, and then in May she spoke at UN headquarters.

The most important outcome was the change in Pakistan's rape law. On 15 November 2006, Pakistan's lower house of Parliament voted to alter its rape laws to move them from religious law to penal code, effectively separating rape from adultery. Parliament also modified the law so that victims are no longer required to produce four witnesses of the assault, and circumstantial and forensic evidence can be used for investigation. The change requires approval of the upper house of Parliament before it becomes law.

Custodial violence includes forced disappearances, torture and cruel or inhuman treatment, and arbitrary executions. Custodial violence against women takes additional forms of rape and other sexual violence. Custodians use rape not only directly against the victim but also against male family members whom they force to witness the rape of women in their family. These scenarios deprive women of their status as victim, because they are merely instruments in the attack on the men (Coomaraswamy 1998).

In U.S. prisons, correctional officers continue to abuse women sexually despite new laws prohibiting it and greater public awareness of the problem (http://www.hrw.org/prisons/united_states.html accessed

26 July 2005). A U.S. government study in December 1999 found pervasive allegations of sexual abuse and misconduct by corrections officers. Criminal prosecutions of abusive staff appeared to increase. Cases since December 1999 included, for example, 11 former guards and a prison official who were indicted on charges of sexually assaulting or harassing 16 female prisoners at a county jail operated by a private corrections company; the conviction of a New Mexico jail guard on federal civil rights charges stemming from the sexual assault of jailed prisoners; the sentencing of a New York jail guard to three years of probation after pleading guilty to sodomizing two female prisoners; and the sentencing of an Ohio jail officer to a four-year prison term for sexually assaulting three female prisoners.

Rape also occurs in public settings like schools, too often perpetrated by teachers or by schoolboys with teachers' complicity. Sexual violence threatens girls' physical safety and psychological welfare, leading to loss of self-esteem, depression, fear for personal safety, anger, and an increased risk of suicide. It may also persuade parents to keep their daughters out of school. In Kenya, a notorious incident occurred on 14 July 1991 when rioting boys killed 19 girls and reportedly raped 71 at St. Kizito School. The principal stated that "The boys never meant any harm against the girls; they just wanted to rape them." The meaning of this statement and the underlying message this principal sent are that it is acceptable for boys to rape girls, though not to kill them. In 1998, the South Africa Demographic and Health Survey assessed the frequency of rape in a nationally representative study of over 11,000 women and found that 153, or 1.6 percent experienced rape before the age of 15. Of these, 33 percent named their schoolteacher as the rapist (PANOS 2003).

In Japan, statutory rape of schoolgirls by their teachers is commonplace; to come forward is to violate a host of powerful social conventions, so victims rarely do so, and only 122 cases were reported in 2001 (French 2003). Victim blaming is usual, and women are taught to be ashamed if they suffer molestation or groping. Talk about the abuse taints the girl for life. The punishment for molestation is dismissal and a one- or two-year prison sentence. Parliamentarian Seiichi Ota said of gang rapists at Tokyo University "the boys are in good shape" and "rather normal" (French 2003).

The Cameroon Association against Child Abuse and Neglect, concerned about violence against schoolgirls, surveyed adolescents in secondary schools in Yaoundé, the capital city: 16 percent had been sexually abused; 73 percent of the abused were girls; and 39 percent of the abused girls were raped—one-third by family members and one-third by school masters (Lobe 2002).

Most rape is private, not public. Intimate partners, relatives, and neighbors inflict most forced sex, not strangers. In Peru, Malaysia, the United States, and many other countries, statistics from the justice system and from studies indicate that 60 to 80 percent of victims know their rapists (PANOS 1998). Gang rapes may be the exception, or perhaps women are more likely to report gang rapes than rapes that occur in the family. Madadgaar, Pakistan's first help line and referral service, reported 520 gang rapes in 2002 and documented all the cases published in newspapers. Madadgaar's research revealed that in most cases the rapists were strangers (475/520) and most rapes occurred in Punjab, an Eastern province of Pakistan on the Indian border (WGNRR 2003c).

Economic and systemic violence

Women run one quarter of the world's households, a figure that varies by country and in some cases comes close to 50 percent. Women who head households experience economic violence through property laws that discriminate against them. Increased ownership of property and land would give more women the collateral they need to obtain credit and run businesses. The list of property regulations that contribute to women's economic marginalization is long. Customary laws, which prevent women from owning land, contradict civil laws, which do not; married couples can count two incomes in getting access to housing but two sisters cannot; married women need their husband's permission to transact property; some inheritance laws give women only half of what a male heir receives; and some married women lose their property when their husbands sell behind their backs (Habitat 1995). The economic violence that structures women's poverty translates into destitution for women and their children. An analysis of the proportion of women in poverty in 10 developing countries[5] found far more poverty for female-headed households and for females, and that in Ghana and Bangladesh women are consistently worse off than men (Quisumbing, Haddad, and Peña 2001).

Women living in informal settlements, a significant proportion of whom head their households, are often worse off, rejected by traditional structures. With no defined socioeconomic status, they cannot integrate in the formal and legal structures of society. Their mobility favors neither regularization nor consolidation of the living environment. "They find themselves locked in a vicious circle: they live in informal settlements because they are marginalised; they are further marginalised because they live in informal settlements" (Habitat 1995, 15).

Unemployment links economic violence to interpersonal violence against women in intricate ways. In societies that emphasize consumerism, a lack of work can deny men the opportunity to achieve ideals of success. Unable to control or economically support their women, unemployed young men trapped in urban slums may reshape ideals of masculinity to emphasize substance abuse, participation in crime, and misogyny, normalizing violence against women. Violence becomes an expression of male vulnerability that stems from unattainable expectations of manhood linked to poverty (Jewkes 2002, 1424, citing the work of Bourgois among Puerto Rican men in New York).

Although violence occurs in all socioeconomic groups, intimate partner violence is more frequent and severe in lower income groups, whether in India, Nicaragua, or the United States (Jewkes 2002). The relation between poverty and abuse is complex and sometimes unexpected: extreme poverty reduces the scope for conflicts about household finance, and financial independence does not always protect women. "Economic inequality within a context of poverty is more important than the absolute level of income or empowerment of a man or woman in a relationship" (Jewkes 2002, 1424).

Economic violence sometimes accompanies interpersonal violence and sometimes follows it, as in Mauritius where S.O.S. Femmes found that after a woman obtained a protection order, the man might stop beating her but increase his economic violence, as well as verbal abuse, threats, and humiliation (Gungaloo 2003). The Mauritian courts do not recognize verbal and economic violence as a breach of the protection order.

In some countries, economic violence takes the form of discrimination against professional women: a glass ceiling can prevent women from pursuing better paying jobs. In Bosnia and Herzegovina most women work in education, health, or social services, but they rarely rise to manage these sectors. No women head hospitals, primary health care centers, or clinics, and no women are deans of educational institutions. The government excludes women from economic decisionmaking posts, and no women hold senior positions in the judiciary, although women dominate the judicial sector. In other words, the public and private sectors exclude women from nearly all influential policymaking jobs (Global Rights 2004). In cases of divorce, women may lose out in the division of property acquired during marriage. Due to inefficiencies in the judiciary, the divorce distribution process may take years, and during that time the husband commonly uses or even sells the property. A husband who sells such jointly held property before the completion of distribution proceedings suffers no meaningful consequences, even when he keeps or diverts all of the profits. This represents a particularly egregious form of economic violence against women, according to women's NGOs (Global Rights 2004).

Political Violence

Political violence intertwines closely with economic violence because political status often determines economic opportunity. Throughout Europe, Roma, Gypsy, and Traveller communities, now the largest ethnic minority within the European Union (EU), lack appropriate documentation such as birth and marriage certificates, residence permits, and identification documents. This lack of papers has created severe problems in accessing social services and in some cases has even led to statelessness. Poverty, poor housing, and persistent discrimination in the provision of health services have resulted in high levels of communicable disease such as tuberculosis and hepatitis and reduced life expectancies. Romani women face double discrimination and correspondingly low levels of access to health, education, and social services. Unemployment rates as high as 80 percent have forced Romani women in several countries including Bulgaria, the Czech Republic, and Slovakia to engage in prostitution. Particularly vulnerable are single mothers, widowed women, and victims of domestic violence. A concomitant problem is the trafficking of Romani women, an unexamined issue that risks feeding widely held stereotypes about Romani criminality (European Commission 2005).

Forced eviction—also known as displacement, ethnic cleansing, expulsion, forced removal, house demolition, land expropriation, population transfer, relocation, resettlement, and slum clearance—is common in conflicts involving competing territorial claims. The coercion is particularly violent for women who are home alone in wartime; lacking the protection of male relatives, women become targets for rape (Farha 2000), causing them to flee. Forced eviction is a form of political violence when the state orders involuntary removal, whether permanent or temporary, with or without the provision of protection or access to legal aid. In addition to the physical violence of eviction, women experience psychological violence as they witness the abduction, torture, and rape of family members and watch the destruction of their livelihoods along with the demolition of their homes. The violence may continue after the eviction if the state fails to give assistance to homeless and landless women; extreme poverty, lack of resources, and loss of family and community may expose women to further assault. "In some cases, women are forced to turn to the sex trade industry in order to survive and in others they have been forced into the industry" (Farha 2000, 75).

Women lack proportionate political representation everywhere: in no country do women have parity in legislatures or ministries. The lack of representation is most severe in some of the world's wealthiest states: it is zero in Brunei, Kuwait, Oman, Qatar, and the United Arab Emirates (UNDP 2004). Where politicians manipulate their power to secure economic opportunity, as in Bosnia and Herzegovina according to the NGO Shadow Report on the implementation of CEDAW and women's human rights, men's near total control over all positions of political power also links directly to gender-based discrimination in the economic arena (Global Rights 2004). Discriminatory practices prevent women from participating equally in the labor market. The result: estimated annual per capita income in Bosnia and Herzegovina is $1,793 for women and $4,135 for men, with women earning an average of 43 cents for every dollar a man earns.

For women living under Muslim law, the most contested political decisions concern family law; in many countries where *shari'a* governs family law, it is the focus of women's calls for reform. On 16 March 2001, nine Moroccan women's associations announced the creation of the Springtime Equality Collective for Reform of the Personal Code (*Collectif Printemps de l'Égalité pour le Réforme du CSP*). The strategies of the collective, which now incorporates 30 women's groups, consist in direct canvassing of the Consultative Commission for the Reform of the *Moudawana*; lobbying the main social and political actors in the country to raise support; and running a media campaign, mobilizing television and the print media, to raise public awareness (*Association Démocratique des Femmes du Maroc* 2003). On 25 January 2004, the Democratic Association of Moroccan Women (*Association Démocratique des Femmes du Maroc*) announced that the government of Morocco adopted a landmark family law supporting women's equality (joint responsibility for the family). Moroccan women now have self-guardianship, a minimum marriage age of 18 years, and new restrictions on polygamy. No longer obligated to obey husbands, women have new rights in divorce (both men and women have the prerogative and can divorce by mutual consent) (www.learningpartnership.org/events/newsalerts/morocco0204.phtml accessed 31 July 2005).

Cultural violence

UNESCO, the United Nations Economic, Social, and Cultural Organization, defines culture in terms of tangible and intangible cultural heritage (http://portal.unesco.org/culture accessed 23 July 2005). Tangible cultural heritage or cultural property includes monuments, religious sites, museums, and libraries. Intangible cultural heritage, sometimes called living cultural heritage, which is pertinent to debates about cultural violence, comprises "the practices, representations, expressions, as well as the knowledge and skills, that communities, groups and, in some cases, individuals recognise as part of their cultural heritage." Intangible cultural heritage is manifested in oral traditions and expressions; performing arts; social practices, rituals and festive events; knowledge and practices concerning nature and the universe; and traditional craftsmanship. Transmitted from generation to generation, and recreated by communities and groups in response to their environment, nature, and historical conditions of existence, intangible cultural heritage "provides people with a sense of identity and continuity, and its safeguarding promotes, sustains, and develops cultural diversity and human creativity." An assumption follows: laws that prevent people from enjoying and perpetuating their intangible cultural heritage constitute acts of cultural violence.

In discussions of women and cultural violence, this broad definition shrinks to a focus on female genital cutting, rape marriages, abduction, and female infanticide. Although culture is widely invoked in debates about women's rights, sometimes female genital cutting is the only example given, as in the resolution on traditional practices affecting the health of women and the girl child adopted by the UN Sub-commission on Human Rights on 17 August 2000; this resolution names only female genital mutilation as a harmful cultural practice. An earlier document from 1994 details a broader list of traditional practices such as early marriage and dowry, the preference for the male child and its implications for the girl child, practices at childbirth, and violence against women including mutilation and bride burning (UN Commission on Human Rights 1994).

Rape marriage, the practice that allows rapists who marry their victims to avoid prosecution, occurs in 12 Latin American countries. In Peru, two groups, CLADEM and DEMUS, demanded repeal of the law. CLADEM (Latin American Committee for the Defense of the Rights of Women) and DEMUS (Defense of Women's Rights, a group of Peruvian lawyers who lobby against violence against women and represent victims of such violence) demanded that rapists be subject to criminal prosecution in all cases (Ms. 1997). Not a new struggle, activists succeeded in 1991 in amending the law to state that if a woman is gang raped, only the rapist who marries her can escape prosecution.

Another type of rape associated with marriage occurs in Ethiopia. Ethiopians define abduction as a form of wife acquisition invoked when a man or woman is unable to marry the person he or she has chosen. In such circumstances, the man forcibly abducts the woman with the help of accomplices and then formalizes the marriage through the mediation of elders. In some cases, the girl arranges the abduction in order to circumvent her family's disapproval of her partner; or a girl's family will arrange the abduction if it is unable to finance the costs of a formal marriage. When abduction entails forced seizure and rape against a young woman's will, community leaders ignore the abuse because the practice is so widely accepted. Abduction is part of a complex social relationship related to family formation and the sustainability of ethnic groups. According to the Regional Women's Affairs Bureau in Southern Nations, Nationalities and Peoples Region, the judicial system treats such cases lightly and slowly, even when they involve violent abduction and rape. Given community opposition to the involvement of the courts in such instances, it is hard for victims to raise a formal complaint, and when the outcome is poor treatment by the system itself, the typical response is to give up (WHO 1999).

Female Genital Cutting

Female genital cutting (FGC) is a traditional practice not related to any single religious or ethnic group. In Ethiopia, Christians, Muslims, and Jews—and people of many different ethnic groups—all performed the ritual. British colonists condemned it in places like Kenya, but only succeeded in entrenching the practice. Feminists like Fran Hoskens and Alice Walker took up the issue, to the consternation of many Southern activists. Calling it female genital mutilation, they seemed to suggest that Southern women could not tackle the issue themselves. Debates continue within Africa over nomenclature (female circumcision, female genital cutting, female genital mutilation) and the best approaches to eradication (Abusharaf and Abdel Halim 2000; Abd El Hadi 2000).

Medicalizing the procedure is one way some countries—Egypt, for example—have avoided the eradication of an operation that the World Health Organization condemns (Abd El Hadi 2000). Others have condemned medicalization: in Sudan, the Sudanese Medical Council banned all types of FGC in March 2003, and the government promised to punish harshly any doctor found violating it by suspending his or her medical license. According to Asma Abdel Halim (personal communication 13 March 2003), a leading Sudanese activist and authority on FGC, it is now incumbent on the Medical Association to start an educational campaign and for doctors and other medical professionals to talk to people about the real dangers of FGC.

But the policies of the successive Sudanese governments have vacillated since outlawing FGC in the 1940s. A public health act banned the practice but "of course [it] was not enforced," and then the regulation disappeared (Asma Abdel Halim, personal communication 13 March 2003). The Sudanese Medical Council felt the need for a public statement because "some doctors are making a fortune of circumcision." Some even limited their practice to circumcision and did not provide any other health service, which left a void in gynecology. Meanwhile, the government started a campaign for Sunna circumcision and had a women gynecologist speak at conferences at women's universities telling everyone how good it is and how it protects from awful diseases. "Isn't it ironic that we need a law to stop the government and not the people?" (Asma Abdel Halim, personal communication 13 March 2003). In March 2007, the Ministry of Social Welfare and Women's and Children's Affairs issued a national policy for the empowerment of women with the goal of eradicating FGC and other harmful practices (Asma Abdel Halim, personal communication 13 March 2003). This policy is a real advance: what measures the government will take to implement it, remains to be seen.

Until recently, the dangers of FGC were largely anecdotal: no scientific study showed the medical consequences. In 2006, WHO published the first evidence of long-term physical harm: severe forms of FGC raise by more than 50 percent the likelihood that a woman or her baby will die in childbirth; lesser forms of FGC raise the chances by 20 percent (WHO 2006). The study of 28,000 women giving birth in hospital covered six African countries.

Thousands of African women have organized to combat FGC, some with international support. A few described here give a sample of the wide range of activity. AMSOPT (*Association Malienne Pour le Suivi et l'Orientation des Pratiques Traditionelles*, a Malian association on traditional practices) is working to curb the practice of genital cutting in Mali, which affects 94 percent of women. In two-thirds of cases, traditional practitioners excise the glands and labia minora, in 17 percent of cases the clitoris is cut, and in 7 percent they practice pharaonic infibulation (excision of clitoris, glands, and labia majora and minora) (Sidibé 1999/2000). Parents prefer to perform the operation in the first month after birth or between the ages of four and five years.

Agnes Pareyio is a 46-year-old Masai woman from Kenya who travels from village to village educating girls about FGC, showing them a plastic female torso with removable vulva. Urging the girls to refuse the cut, Pareyio shows a whole vulva, then one without a clitoris, and then an infibulated vulva. In 2000 she met Eve Ensler who funds her V-Day foundation with royalties from her successful play, *The Vagina Monologues*; the V-Day foundation gave Pareyio a jeep, a cell phone, and $65,000 for a "safe house" for girls escaping FGC (Baumgardner 2002). The Kenyan campaign to eradicate FGC brings together 67 organizations that are also promoting an alternative rite of passage for 12- to 13-year-old girls (Ben-Ari 2003).

Rainbo, the creation of Nahid Toubia a Sudanese physician, is a non-profit organization working on women's reproductive health and sexual rights that focuses on awareness and prevention of the practice of female genital cutting. Rainbo runs a resource center and provides technical support to international agencies working in FGC programming and policy development; it participates in interagency working group meetings with UN agencies, donor agencies, private foundations, research and technical organizations, and NGOs; and it supports innovative projects developed by local African organizations working to eradicate FGC through a grant program. Sauti Yetu (which is Swahili for "Our Voice," www.sautiyetu.org) split off from Rainbo to address the reproductive health concerns (including FGC) of African immigrants living in the United States.

Tostan is a Senegalese nongovernmental organization that works to eradicate FGC through yearlong programs of education about human rights and women's health, especially the risks and dangers of genital cutting. Tostan does not instruct people to stop the practice, but after following the program they often decide to abandon it; so far a total of 1,993 villages, representing nearly 40 percent of the 5,000 communities that practice FGC have made public declarations to end the practice (www.tostan.org/.news-jan_07.htm accessed 6 April 2007).

On 11 July 2003, the African Union adopted the Maputo Protocol to the African Charter on Human and Peoples' Rights on the Rights of Women in Africa. Advancing the human rights of African women through creative, substantive, and detailed language, the new Protocol covers a broad range of women's human rights issues. For the first time in international law, it explicitly calls for the legal prohibition of female genital mutilation; it also stipulates a prohibition on the amelioration or preservation of harmful practices such as the medicalization and para-medicalization of female genital mutilation and scarification, in order to effect a total elimination of such practices. By October 2005, the required 15 African countries had ratified the protocol bringing the commitment to defend the rights of women and their physical integrity into force. Meanwhile, 14 African countries have banned or criminalized FGC.[6]

Wartime Violence

War exposes women to all of the types of violence discussed above. Because a series of deliberate policy decisions produces wartime rape, sexual violence against women in wartime is categorically different from rape in "peaceful" societies. Rape in wartime is often a collective act; perpetrators act collectively and choose their victims because they are members of a political, ethnic, or religious group.

West African women meeting in 1998 to discuss women and war distinguished between explicit and implicit violence (Turshen and Alidou 2000). Explicit violence includes: systematic rape used to dishonor and humiliate, not just women, but the enemy; forced pregnancy, which leaves the enemy's marker; shooting women through the vagina to render them infertile and to end the enemy's ability to reproduce; gang rape; mutilation; cutting open the pregnant womb and killing the fetus; sexual slavery and forced labor; and forcing children to witness their mother's rape. Implicit violence includes abandoning women to fend for themselves and their children; police and military harassment and intimidation; the opportunistic violence of bandits, rapists, and thieves; social and governmental institutional discrimination (for example, denial of access to media); forced prostitution; the silence of leaders on increased prostitution, which makes them accomplices; looting and the dispossession of women, which leaders protect and vindicate; politicians' and media's verbal abuse and disrespect of women; denial of access to resources and restricting access to women of certain political affiliations; sexual harassment of women who join the armed forces; denial of abortion on demand in cases of pregnancy resulting from systematic rape; rejection of women victims of systematic rape; rejection of children conceived in rape; imprisonment of women of all ages without recourse to justice or outside assistance; and lack of research or reliable documentation on the state of women before, during, and after war—this amounts to a conspiracy of leaders to maintain silence.

Several intergovernmental organizations have taken up the issue of wartime rape. The examples detailed here concern Yugoslavia, Rwanda, Peru, and East Timor. The International Criminal Tribunal on the Former Yugoslavia (established in 1993) and the International Criminal

Tribunal on Rwanda (established in 1995) have changed the legal status of wartime rape from an expected, if not accepted, accompaniment of war to a crime of war. The mass rapes that took place in the former Yugoslavia, particularly those in Bosnia and Herzegovina, were the first to be brought before an international court. The statutes of both courts singled out rape as a crime against humanity, an act committed as part of a widespread or systematic attack against a civilian population on national, political, ethnic, racial, or religious grounds. The International Criminal Tribunal on Rwanda was the first to prosecute and find a defendant guilty under the new statute.

The Women's Rights Project of Human Rights Watch and Americas Watch reported in 1993 that Peruvian government security forces and the Shining Path (*Sendero Luminoso*) insurgency used violence, including rape and murder, against noncombatant women as a tactic of warfare. Soldiers and police routinely raped women with impunity, while the Shining Path often murdered women to punish, intimidate, or coerce them or as part of their efforts to achieve broader political ends. In judicial proceedings for the rare accusation of rape, the judge took into consideration a woman's "honor," age, and sexual past. There is little national redress for women victims of sexual violence in Peru, so lawyers have filed some cases before the Inter-American Court of Human Rights. A decision of the Inter-American Court found that Peru's security forces had arbitrarily detained, tortured, and raped Maria Elena Loayza and ordered her release. On 2 October 1997, the Peruvian Government released the university teacher, who had been imprisoned since 1993 (Coomaraswamy 1998).

After voting for independence in 1999, East Timor experienced extreme violence; the Indonesian military and the local militias it commanded destroyed the country and raped the women (Mydans 2001). Fokupers, Timor-Leste Women's Communication Forum founded in 1997, investigated the assaults on women and found that militia members and soldiers connived to abduct women, share them, or forcibly take them across the border to West Timor where they raped the women daily and forced them to perform household chores (www.hivos.nl accessed 17 July 2004). The United Nations compiled cases against the rapists for the Commission for Reception, Truth, and Reconciliation in Timor-Leste (CAVR). On 22 April 2003, CAVR held a public hearing on women and conflict in Timor-Leste to reveal human rights violations and to educate the public about reasons for and patterns of human rights abuses and about women's rights. Fokupers is one of the East Timorese women's NGOs working on the empowerment of women from the perspective of women's human rights. Some others are the Popular Organization of Timorese Women (OMPT); FRETILIN's women's organization, established in 1975 to promote the emancipation of women in all aspects of life; the Timor-Leste Women's Network (REDE Feto), a network of civil society organizations committed to the advancement of women in Timor-Leste; Timor-Leste Women Against Violence (ETWAVE), which collected data in 1998 from the victims of violence; and the Women's Caucus (Caucus Feto), a nonpartisan civil society organization. Despite the difficulties of accessing and supporting people throughout the country under these circumstances, the UN's involvement in Timor-Leste was a success; the strong inclusion of gender components in the mission's activities has ensured that women are involved in the reconstruction of Timor-Leste and that they fully participate in the independent Timorese future (UNIFEM 2005).

Although rape in wartime and peacetime are categorically different, researchers have noted an increase in rape in the aftermath of war, in both defeated communities and among victors (Meintjes, Pillay, and Turshen 2002). In the aftermath of war, violence and militarism become entrenched in many societies. We know little about the effects of war on the people who wage it, the relation to civilians of military personnel trained to kill, the role of military institutional values in creating ideals of violent masculinity and virulent misogyny, and the relation of the militarization of society to the epidemic of violence against women. We do know that men are responsible for 90 per cent of all physical violence and that men's violence against women is rooted in male roles and masculinities (Breines, Connell, and Eide 2000).

These questions are more acute and critical in the United States since September 11th 2001 and the U.S.-led invasions of Afghanistan and Iraq; men in uniform (police, firefighters, soldiers) are glorified, worshipped as heroes, and pitied as victims. What of the women they batter, rape, torture, and kill? An analysis of five deaths at Fort Bragg, Fayetteville, NC, in 2002 revealed that all five women were victims of domestic violence—beatings, stabbings, shootings, and strangulations—perpetrated by their husbands, who were accused of their murders (Elliston and Lutz 2003). Three of the soldiers had served in Special Operations, which with Delta Force is the army's toughest unit and among the last to include women. The military's culture institutionalizes the promotion of violence and fails to address its effect on home life: there is little "actual dialogue about the potential ties between military values and domestic violence" (Elliston and Lutz 2003, 28). Survivors Take Action against Abuse by Military Personnel is a national network of counseling groups based in Ohio: they point out that the military fails to see the many military scandals of the last 15 years as part of the epidemic of violent abuse by men in the military, including rape of female (and some male) soldiers and civilians, lesbian and gay bashing, and brutal hazing rituals (Lutz and Elliston 2002).

Mary Beth Loucks-Sorrell, interim director of the North Carolina Coalition Against Domestic Violence, a statewide umbrella group based in Durham, said she is convinced, based on years of experience, that "women partnered with soldiers face disproportionate risks of domestic abuse" (Elliston and Lutz 2003, 26). The Miles Foundation, an advocacy group for victims of military domestic violence, found that rates of domestic violence in the military rose to 25.6 per 1,000 soldiers in 1996 from 18.6 per 1,000 in 1990. Rates in the military are two to five times higher than in the civilian population (Butterfield 2002). One army-funded study found that reports of severe aggression against spouses ran more than three times higher among army families than among civilian ones in 1998 (Lutz and Elliston 2002).

The link between domestic abuse and a culture of violence, in which men use force to resolve personal as well as political problems, is also the concern of the Israeli Coalition of Women for Peace.[7] They note that since the beginning of the second *intifada* in 2001, Israel has seen more rape, more killing of women by their male partners, and more violence in schools by children. "The overlap between the 'war on terror' and increased violence in the streets, homes, and schools is no coincidence" (Svirsky 2004).

Refugee Women

The United Nations distinguishes between refugees, who cross international borders to escape conflict, and internally displaced people who move from their homes in the conflict area to some other part of the country in search of safety. Like male refugees, women need adequate protection against forcible return to their countries of origin and other forms of violence like armed attacks. Outside of their own countries, women may be unable or unwilling to access the protection that their own governments should provide. Refugee women and girls also need special protection for problems related to their gender, such as sexual exploitation, physical abuse, and sexual discrimination in the distribution of goods and services. Common risks faced by women and children before they reach a place of refuge include the use of rape and sexual abuse as weapons of war and demands for sex in exchange for safe passage.

The Women's Rights Project of Human Rights Watch and Africa Watch reported in 1993 on sexual abuse of Somali women in refugee camps in Kenya. Unidentified armed bands and former Somali military men attacked women as old as 50 and girls as young as 4, night or day on the outskirts of the camps where women and girls went to herd goats or collect firewood. The bands gang raped the women, and robbed, beat, knifed, or shot them. To penetrate infibulated women, they cut or tore the women's vaginal opening. Many of these women suffered rape in Somalia before fleeing to Kenya. The majority of rapes also involved looting and robbery, even of the victims' refugee food ration cards and kitchen utensils. A number of women who ran successful trading businesses in the camps became targets and were forced to pay protection money to Kenyan camp guards or the Somali militia and bandits (Gardner and El Bushra 2004).

Somali refugee women made the headlines in the 1990s; today it is Sudanese women. In Darfur, a large region of six million people in western Sudan, government forces and allied militias continue to kill thousands and displace tens of thousands of people living in rural areas. As of March 2007, some 2.2 million displaced people remained in camps within Darfur or elsewhere in Sudan and more than 230,000 Darfur refugees remained in Chad. "Rape and sexual violence have been used to terrorize and uproot rural communities in Darfur," said Peter Takirambudde, Africa director of Human Rights Watch (HRW 2005). Soldiers or Janjawid militiamen raped thousands of women, sometimes in public, and took many as sexual slaves. Women continue to be raped outside of camps for internally displaced persons (IDPs).

An 18-year-old woman described how after an attack on Mukjar in January [2004] about 45 women were taken from the village by soldiers and militiamen wearing military uniform and raped. She was raped by six men and given to a soldier who kept her in sexual slavery for one month in Nyala and then took her to Khartoum, where she remained for two months before escaping. The soldier was under investigation at the end of the year.

In August [2004], armed men in uniform, apparently from militias, reportedly raped three teenage girls gathering wood outside Ardamata IDP camp. The women reported the rape to the police who sent them for a medical examination but subsequently dropped the case.

In April [2005], a UN mission described how 1,700 IDPs, whose villages had been burnt, were confined to the town of Kailek in

Shattaya district, West Darfur, without access to food or water. The town was encircled by the Janjawid who would take women to rape at night and subject men to forced labour. (Amnesty International www.amnesty.org accessed 29 July 2005)

The response of Sudanese authorities has exacerbated an already appalling situation. Human Rights Watch documented how authorities in Bindisi, West Darfur, harassed and detained pregnant girls and women, many of whom had become pregnant as a result of rape. Rather than investigating the crimes, the authorities often accuse the victims, threatening them with charges of fornication if they do not pay a fine. Under Sudanese law, women who bring rape charges may face prosecution: a pregnant unmarried woman who cannot prove she has been raped can be charged with adultery, a capital crime. Proof requires the testimony of four witnesses (Hoge 2005).

The Chadian authorities imprisoned some women living in the refugee camps in Chad for trying to collect firewood outside the camps; Chadian inmates then raped the women in jail. Human Rights Watch documented 10 cases of women and girls from Farchana camp who were imprisoned in such circumstances in January 2005. In some refugee camps in Chad, police and male residents have coerced women and girls to provide "sexual services" in exchange for "protection" (HRW 2005).

Torture

Darfur security forces, military intelligence, and police routinely torture detainees (Amnesty International www.amnesty.org accessed 29 July 2005). In August 2004, the Positive Security arrested 12 people from Mellit, North Darfur state, and tortured them to make them confess to fabricating a videotape showing rapes. The security men beat with a belt, kicked, and punched four women, Mariam Mohamed Dinar, Su'ad Ali Khalil, Su'ad al-Nur Abdel Rahman, and Fatma Rahma. With pincers they pulled out the nails of Mariam Mohamed Dinar. Men arrested at the same time were also reportedly tortured. The charges were later dropped and all were released in November 2004.

Torturing women and men with sexual violence deliberately degrades and humiliates the victims (Moser and Clarke 2001). Evidence shows that certain forms of violence are specific to women and that the sexualization of women's torture has gender-specific effects: sexual abuse has special consequences for women, such as the risk of pregnancy, miscarriage, forced abortion, or sterilization, and of sexually transmitted diseases that may lead to sterility; and where rape and sexual abuse stigmatize and ostracize the victim, she may be unable to return to her community and family (United Nations 2004).

The World Health Organization convened an expert committee meeting on torture in 1977; its report made no mention of gendered treatment of prisoners. Definitions of torture did not include rape until 1992, when the UN Special Rapporteur on Torture clearly defined rape as a form of torture (Coomaraswamy 1998). War-related sexual violence, although a recurrent phenomenon throughout history, became a crime against humanity only in 1993. The United Nations acknowledged that systematic rape is used as a practice of torture to terrorize and humiliate selected ethnic groups. The International Criminal Tribunal for Rwanda held in the Akayesu judgment that "[s]exual violence was an integral part of the process of destruction, specifically targeting Tutsi women and specifically contributing to their destruction and to the destruction of the Tutsi group as a whole" (ICTR 1998). The International Criminal Tribunal for the Former Yugoslavia defined sexual violence as torture, inhuman punishment, great suffering, or serious injury (Coomaraswamy 1998).

U.S. Attorney General Alberto Gonzales has said that torture may be legally construed as acts that bring the prisoner near the pain of death. In the sixth report submitted to the UN General Assembly in 2004, the UN Special Rapporteur on Torture drew attention to this attempt to circumvent the absolute and non-derogable[8] nature of the prohibition of torture and other forms of cruel, inhuman, or degrading treatment or punishment (United Nations 2004). The United Nations' definition makes the United States liable for prosecution under international law.

> Legal arguments of necessity and self-defence, invoking domestic law, have recently been put forward, aimed at providing a justification to exempt officials suspected of having committed or instigated acts of torture against suspected terrorists from criminal liability. While being aware of the threats posed by terrorism and recognizing the duty of States to protect their citizens and the security of the State against such threats, the Special Rapporteur would like to reiterate that the absolute nature of the prohibition of torture and other forms of ill-treatment means that no exceptional circumstances whatsoever, whether a state of war or a threat of war, internal political instability or any other public emergency, may be invoked as a justification for torture. (United Nations 2004, para. 14)

The women soldiers stationed at Guantánamo Bay who participate in interrogations may be liable for their degrading treatment of prisoners: the U.S. military has turned them into "sex workers," performing "pseudo lap-dances," smearing fake menstrual blood on detainees, rubbing up against prisoners, and touching them "inappropriately." The *New York Times* calls this "the exploitation and debasement of women serving in the United States military," a violation of American moral values (Editorial, 15 July 2005).

The Costs of Violence

A rule of silence in the general population and even among some torture survivors surrounds the phenomenon of torture. The silence creates misunderstanding or reinforces a sense of loneliness, and children may feel the effects of their parents' torture even if they did not witness it. These are some of the psychological costs of violence that have been calculated in dollar equivalencies.

Intimate partner violence costs the United States about $12.6 billion each year; it costs Nicaragua $32.7 million (1.6 percent of GDP) and Chile $1.73 billion (2 percent of GDP) (Waters et al. 2004). The figures for all forms of interpersonal violence, including youth violence and gun-related violence, child abuse and neglect, and workplace violence, are much higher: the United States spends about $300 billion per year on violence-related problems; and economic losses from all types of violence in El Salvador total 24.9 percent of its GDP. Costs include legal and medical costs, the costs of policing and incarceration, and the losses to earnings and productivity. Interpersonal violence diverts billions of dollars away from education, health, housing, and social security.

Around 1,400 people die of interpersonal violence each day and many more are injured (Waters et al. 2004). Nancy Cardia, University of Sao Paulo, Brazil, calls the WHO report on the economic dimensions of interpersonal violence "very important" because it looks at a long-neglected issue. She believes governments respond better to economic arguments than to ethical ones, so WHO's report is particularly useful; but Cardia doubts that recognition of the problem will be translated into good prevention programs (*The Lancet* 2004). Patricia Omidian who has worked on violence against women in Afghanistan and Pakistan adds that although there is an interest in the prevention of interpersonal violence in the global North, in the global South the issue receives scant attention. Governments rarely fund domestic violence services. Omidian said, "In some countries, such as Pakistan and Afghanistan, services for women trying to escape violence are usually referred to the courts, which act against the woman by putting her in prison where she and her children are at risk for further violence" (*The Lancet* 2004, 2058).

Throughout the literature on the costs of violence, psychological costs greatly outweigh the direct costs of violence (Waters et al. 2004). The Illinois Coalition against Sexual Assault, an advocacy group, calculated that the average sexual assault results in $110,000 in costs to the victim, including $500 in medical care, $2,400 in mental health services, $2,200 in lost productivity, and $104,900 in undiscounted pain and suffering (Waters et al. 2004). Battering has long-term negative health consequences for survivors, even after the abuse has ended. These effects can manifest as poor health status, poor quality of life, and high use of health services.

Prevention is inexpensive and the savings are significant. The 1994 Violence against Women Act in the United States resulted in an estimated net benefit of $16.4 billion, including $14.8 billion in averted victim's costs. A separate analysis showed that providing shelters for victims of domestic violence resulted in a benefit to cost ratio between 6.8 and 18.4 (Waters et al. 2004).

Data from several studies suggest that socioeconomic inequalities drive the effect of other factors such as poverty, race, and geographical location on violence. These studies argue for the position that inequality rather than absolute deprivation produced by poverty is a risk factor for interpersonal violence. Data for homicides from 31 nations on the relationship between homicide, inequality, and economic development indicate that inequality is a better predictor of violence than economic development. Homicide rates decrease with development, independent of inequality, but increasing inequality predisposes to more lethal violence (Waters et al. 2004). Note that the WHO study makes no mention of sexism or sustained discrimination against women. The authors consider neither the legal framework nor the social context of violence against women, just as Therborn (2004) fails to consider violence against women in his sociological study of the family.

CHAPTER SIX

Women's Reproductive Rights

Technology has transformed reproductive health care and choices, but with different consequences for women belonging to powerful groups and women in subordinated positions. Racism and class prejudice distort women's experiences; disadvantaged women of color everywhere are disproportionately the targets of population programs; and the state has too often manipulated technology in the interests of political objectives. Technology can be liberating; technologies for contraception and the treatment of infertility can expand women's choices and enhance their ability to control their lives. Technology can also limit women's decision-making and can be abused and abusive in the hands of policymakers and patriarchs. The abuse of technology leads to fetal sex selection, the commodification of body parts, and infertility treatment as a profitable business. Technology, and the commercial interests vested in its production and diffusion, conflicts with medical and epidemiological research into such reproductive health issues as the environmental causes of breast cancer. Moreover, the routine use of breast implants for breast reconstruction and enhancement raises the issue of what counts as body modification, what as body mutilation.

This chapter follows the arguments of women's health movements around the conflicts between, on the one hand, the reproductive rights of individual women and the social groups they belong to and, on the other hand, religious dogma and national and international population control plans. Some women's groups are asking whether they really benefit from the new reproductive technologies, raising questions related to gender, ethnicity, and biology. The issues of new reproductive technologies for the treatment of infertility raised in this chapter are not restricted to advanced industrial societies; in vitro fertilization, for example, is on the increase in India and there are eight centers in sub-Saharan Africa (WHO 2003b).

Women's Reproductive Health and Rights

Population control to change aggregate population characteristics has dominated reproductive health policies since the Second World War. The policies encompass pronatalist, eugenic, and antinatalist strategies. Planning families to limit their size through the use of birth control became a question of economic and national security at the end of Second World War, as colonial empires in the Middle East, Asia, the Caribbean, and Africa slipped from the grasp of Europe and the United States. Independence exposed the depredations of imperialism to world scrutiny, and self-rule inaugurated a rise in population that the shrinking European powers found threatening. A national and international issue, rates of population growth obsessed policymakers and drove the development of new contraceptive technology, capturing basic scientific and pharmaceutical research. In a climate of intense competition between superpowers promoting radically different ideologies of development in the Third World, a newly secularizing Europe joined the United States, now a world power, in persuading the United Nations first to address and eventually to adopt population control as the leading measure of economic development. The trend to focus on population control climaxed in the 1970s in a series of dramatic events: the proclamation of the New International Economic Order (NIEO) by the nonaligned states in 1972; the emergent power of OPEC (the Organization of Petroleum Exporting Countries) in 1973, putting the Middle East in the center of resource struggles; the punishing sterilization camps in India, a policy that brought down the government of Indira Gandhi (Rao 1999); and the World Population Conference in Bucharest in 1974, at which the Marxist analysis of economic underdevelopment (as elaborated in the NIEO) clashed with the capitalist program for population control. Also at this conference, China—a country that the United Nations admitted in 1972, replacing Taiwan in the permanent seat on the Security Council—changed sides on the population debates; the Chinese government later announced the adoption of the one child policy. In response to these and other challenges (not least the 1975 Vietnamese victory in the American war), the Northern powers introduced the neoliberal policies of globalization and structural adjustment.

In 1975 the international women's movement stepped onto the world stage in the International Year of the Woman, followed by the first International Tribunal on Crimes against Women, held in Brussels in March 1976, and the International Decade for Women, 1976–1985. Women's groups brought different priorities to the discussion of sexual and reproductive health, reflecting the varied stages of economic and social development of their countries, the relative influence of conservative religious factions, and the political and legal status of women.

In Latin America, women's health movements emphasized quality reproductive and sexual health services in the face of religious and state oppression and in the context of citizenship needs.[1] In Asia women were concerned with population control and coercion, maternal mortality, the health of the girl child and all forms of violence against women. Activists in Africa were concerned with poverty and survival issues, maternal mortality and morbidity, sexually transmitted diseases and HIV/AIDS. European and North American women focused on autonomy and expression, the medicalization of reproductive health, and the rising cost of services. Middle Eastern women were concerned with access and rights to holistic reproductive health care throughout the life cycle. Central and Eastern European women focused on public health, gender equality, and women's rights issues (Global Health Watch 2005).

In the 1980s women's groups began advocating a shift from population control objectives to broad reproductive and sexual health programs. Women debated the universal applicability of the concept of reproductive rights and the importance of sensitivity to the individual needs and differences of countries in the global South. How to refine the meaning of "choice" in relation to reproductive technologies is a recurrent theme (Garcia-Moreno and Claro 1994).

Women everywhere were finding that the exclusive focus on population control was destructive of women's health and health services. Family planning programs—always concentrated on women's bodies with scant attention paid to men—absorbed almost all of the available resources; they took the form of vertical (single-purpose) services that distorted primary health, school health, and occupational health programs, drained health budgets, and reassigned health personnel to fertility control.[2] Health economists and health planners designed programs for the reproductive years, neglecting childhood, adolescence, and old age; they evinced little interest in women's needs beyond medical attention in pregnancy and childbirth, although infectious diseases were still the cause of two-thirds of all women's deaths in many underdeveloped countries. As a result of this exclusive focus on lowering the birth rate, governments did not invest in basic public health measures that could have improved women's health and made their lives less burdensome. The Asia-Pacific Resource and Research Center for Women (ARROW) found in a review of seven Southeast Asian countries that "hardly any data and information [were] available on the prevalence of reproductive cancers, reproductive tract infections and STDs, [or] the extent of service availability. In fact the only reliable data in all countries was on contraceptive use" (Abdullah 2003, 34). The Indian family planning program acquired the nature of a black hole that sucked in the entire health services, observed the medical activist, Debabar Banerji (1992). Population control programs were not even particularly successful in India; despite millions poured into plans and some of the most coercive strategies, "the family planning programme, one of the largest public health programmes in the world, has quite simply failed to take off" (Rao 1999, 95).

Reproduction as a Woman's Right

How to frame the demand for reproductive health care has preoccupied women's health movements since the 1970s. A fundamental premise of women's health movements is that women's health and empowerment are goals in their own right, not means to reduce fertility. An ongoing dilemma for feminists is how to campaign for access to birth control and reproductive health services without seeming to collude with proponents of population control. The traditional emphasis on maternal and child health, a staple of public health and missionary medicine all over the world, implied a focus on the child or, at best, the mother-child dyad; it carried the sense that the mother was the vessel for the child, that the child was the more valued of the two, and that the provision of maternal and child health services was a cost effective means to improve child welfare. Many women's groups choose human rights as their framework, shifting the focus to the woman; human rights give activists an accepted body of law to use in their criticisms of population control programs.

Women's groups make an important distinction between meeting needs and fulfilling rights. The rights approach reformulates needs as ethical and legal norms—implying the duty of those in power to provide all the means necessary to meet women's needs. Bearers of rights can make official claims as citizens when governments argue that they lack the necessary resources. As individuals and groups, women are also in a stronger position to become part of the decisionmaking process and defend themselves against other powerful influences including religious and fundamentalist groups. As well they can stand against the macroeconomic or neo-Malthusian agendas that perpetuate racial, ethnic, class, and gender inequities (UNRISD 2000). Many women of color who are activists for reproductive rights in the United States find the human rights framework one of the best ways to articulate and advance their rights because this framework links together civil, political, economic, sexual, and social rights. Resisting population control while simultaneously claiming their right to bodily self-determination, including the right to contraception and abortion or to have children, is at the heart of their struggles for reproductive control (Silliman et al. 2004). ARROW, based in Kuala Lumpur, is an example of a nongovernmental organization that uses a rights frame; ARROW advocates that countries in the region adopt a gender and rights approach to women's sexual and reproductive health rights and needs by providing accessible, affordable, comprehensive health and reproductive services as well as population policies and programs (Abdullah 2003).

Women's organizations everywhere in the South insist that reproductive rights must be set in a broad context. They contend that the prospect of fulfilling women's individual rights in a generally hostile economic and social climate is almost nil. A number of international networks make this case forcefully, notably Development Alternatives with Women for a New Era (DAWN), one of the most influential networks of women activists from all regions of the South. DAWN argues that women can achieve reproductive rights only in a supportive environment that allows adequate housing, education, employment, property rights, and legal equality, as well as freedom from physical abuse, harassment, and all forms of gender-based violence (www.dawnnet.org accessed 10 April 2007). Reproductive rights require civil and political rights: legal recognition and protection in the courts, freedom from repressive religious and traditional codes that constrain choice, and freedom from domestic violence and forced pregnancy. Reproductive rights also require economic and social rights: reliable and affordable maternal and child health services, access to safe contraception and follow-up care, and adequate nutrition to avoid a wide range of risks (UNRISD 2000).

Birth control policies, which are ostensibly part of planning national development and economic growth, are—at the individual level—about who has how many children: race, ethnicity, and class are the determinants in the global South as well as the North. Some governments (China, India) are anxious to lower birth rates (some under pressure from the World Bank and donors)—either the average national rate or the rate in selected communities (for example, France wants to lower the immigrant birthrate, and apartheid South Africa wanted to lower the black birth rate). These governments prescribe when and at what age women should have children; how many children women should have; and whether some should have no children (through sterilization campaigns in India or the United States) or no more children (through punitive welfare policies in China or the United States).

Governments that adopt strict policies to control the number of births reason that their population is already too large in relation to acres of arable land and rates of socioeconomic progress. Fertility control also enables states to regulate the workforce by determining the numbers of workers entering labor markets (and working women, they find, have fewer children). Some countries use population control programs in conjunction with a range of policies that affect birth rates: taxes and income supports, family allowances and benefits, food and housing subsidies, health and education policies, laws on age at first marriage, legal controls on sex between unmarried couples, equal opportunity laws, and so on. In its population policy announced in February 2000, the Government of India endorsed voluntary and informed choice in family planning programs, but a number of states have implemented restrictions. The state of Maharashtra refuses nutritional supplements to poor tribal women with a third pregnancy, limits grain allotments to the first two children, and disbars candidates with more than two children from standing in many local elections (Hartmann 2001). Six states have laws mandating a two-child norm for members of village councils, and some states are offering incentives like pay raises or access to land or housing to government servants who choose sterilization after one or two children. A national bill limiting members of Parliament and state legislators to two children would affect low-caste members and women, for whom the 1992 constitutional amendment set aside seats in an effort to democratize government (Waldman 2003).

Coercive family planning programs usually impose limits on family size but some aim to compel couples to bear more children than they want by banning abortion and contraception. Pronatalist programs like the one in Romania under the regime of Nicolae Ceausescu (1965–1989), which denied women access to contraception and abortion, are coercive in this way. In 1966 Romania overturned its previously liberal abortion policy, ostensibly to increase population in the name of promoting socioeconomic development. In 1985 the government tightened the prohibition on abortion and all but banned contraceptives; it forced women to undergo gynecological exams and monitored pregnancies to delivery. The results were dramatic: Romania had the second highest infant mortality rate in Europe; their maternal mortality rate was eight times higher than next highest in Europe; 9,452 deaths related to abortion occurred over the 24 years of Ceausescu's regime; 20,000 women were hospitalized for complications of unsafe, illegal abortions; and unknown numbers of orphans were placed in state orphanages (Kligman 1995). Pronatalist programs are once again common in Eastern and Central Europe where governments have adopted new prohibitions on abortion.

Fundamentalist readings of various religious texts—Buddhist, Christian, Hindu, Jewish, and Muslim—lead to ideological opposition to birth control, adding another dimension to issues of race and class. All religions incorporate an important element of social control, have strong precepts on masculine and feminine conduct, and impose sanctions on unacceptable, nonconforming behavior. Gender roles of women and men are at the core of contested understandings of sexuality. Although the Christian right[3] in the United States talks in terms of the social roles of women and men, the upshot of their position is control of women's labor in the home and for the family. Their agenda extends to the racial and ethnic hierarchy of women in the labor force and the control of the size, racial, and ethnic composition of the labor force. By adopting welfare laws that dictate how many children poor women can raise, the division between fulltime and part-time mothers becomes a class, racial, and ethnic split. For many women workers the struggle for reproductive rights is the struggle to have healthy children and maintain them in economic health, a struggle that encompasses working in nontoxic environments and gaining paid family leave after birth or adoption (Stein 2002).

Women Mobilize for Their Rights

Building on the International Decade for Women, women's health movements organized around reproductive rights. In 1984, the International Contraception, Abortion and Sterilization Campaign (ICASC)[4] organized the Fourth International Women and Health Meeting, the International Tribunal on Reproductive Rights, in Amsterdam; women from the South and North testified about reproductive abuses, and reproductive rights emerged as a major issue (Garcia-Moreno and Claro 1994). For the UN Conference on the Environment and Development held in Rio de Janeiro in 1992, WEDO (1992) organized the World Women's Congress for a Healthy Planet in Miami in 1991; the Congress produced the Women's Action Agenda, which (among other things) decried blaming women's fertility rates for environmental degradation, pointing instead to industrial and military pollutants, toxic wastes, and economic systems that exploit and misuse nature and people. Action Agenda 21 condemned attempts to deprive women of reproductive freedom and demanded women-centered, women-managed, comprehensive reproductive health care and family planning. The 1993 Vienna World Conference on Human Rights, at which women's groups held a tribunal and lobbied hard for the recognition of women's human rights, reaffirmed a woman's right to accessible and adequate health care and the widest range of family planning services.

Also in 1993, the Committee on Women, Population and the Environment issued the Statement on Women, Population and Environment: Call for a New Approach (CWPE 1995), which over 365 individuals and organizations endorsed. More than 2,400 individuals and organizations— including grassroots organizations, professional associations, and academic institutions—from over 105 countries and across a range of sectors like health, family planning, environment, and development signed the Women's Declaration on Population Policies (Garcia-Moreno and Claro 1994). The Women's Declaration and DAWN's Population Policies and Reproductive Rights Project are calls to reconsider debt repayment, international trade agreements, and structural adjustment programs, and to provide adequate funds and support in government budgets for health services and other basic needs. Southern women believe that changes in these policies are essential for the lasting achievement of health and rights. Neoliberal economic fundamentalism, no less than religious or ethnic fundamentalism, is intent on dismantling the reproductive rights agenda, and the consequences for women are loss of livelihood and economic insecurity as well as loss of control over their life choices and bodies (Harcourt 2003).

Despite solidarity on fundamental points of reproductive rights, substantial diversity emerged in the movement on matters of substance as well as political strategy, both across and within countries. The debates among feminists who work inside family planning and population agencies and feminists outside the population establishment reflect that diversity. Feminists who work as service providers, researchers, and managers attempt to improve the quality of family planning services, expand services to broaden reproductive health care, and provide information and services to young people and others excluded from programs. They also work to transform policies to meet women's needs, secure financial support for women's health groups, and include women's health advocates in the work of their agencies. Feminists outside the population establishment oppose population policies, think that collaboration with the establishment inevitably leads to cooptation, consider population programs inimical to women's interests, and believe in taking action to dismantle them rather than trying to modify them to meet women's needs (Garcia-Moreno and Claro 1994).[5]

The Program of Action that emerged from the Cairo International Conference on Population and Development in 1994 endorsed women's vision of reproductive rights and health and moved away from demographic targets and a narrow preoccupation with family planning. Population agencies and aid programs agreed to base population and development strategies on women's empowerment, gender equality, and equity. The Cairo Program of Action also endorsed market-friendly policies that, in practice, hamper the achievement of women's reproductive rights. Although the Cairo Program recognizes the devastating impact of structural adjustment on health and the difficulties experienced in planned economies transiting to market capitalism, its implementation chapters revert to market-oriented policies that widen disparities in income, mortality, and morbidity. The Cairo Program urges governments to reintroduce user fees to improve the cost-effectiveness, cost-recovery, and quality of services; it asks them to promote the role of the private sector in production, distribution, and delivery of reproductive health services and family planning commodities; and it calls for a review of legal, regulatory, and import policies that unnecessarily prevent or restrict the greater involvement of the private sector (UNRISD 2000).

If the Cairo Program gave rights while it took away the promise of achievement, the post-Cairo decade saw both the enhanced legitimacy of women's organizations and the determined opposition of conservative forces. With the support of the international community, women's organizations pressured their governments to follow through on their Cairo commitments. At the same time the Vatican and its allies sought to undo the agreements reached in Cairo. The inclusion of reproductive rights and health in the population control agenda also reopened divisions within women's health movements. Radical women's organizations felt that the new rhetoric would not necessarily change anything in practice (UNRISD 2000). Some women's groups believed that population control agencies were coopting the term "reproductive rights," using it as a cover for coercive family planning programs. Women working in Africa deem new concerns with maternal mortality as corresponding to the population control agenda (De Koninck 1998). Morsy (1995, 173) writes, "the selective focus on maternal mortality appears to be a medicalized form of fertility regulation." Some groups see the limitations of framing women's health as reproductive rights, narrowing the focus to women's childbearing capacity: they want rights vested in women as citizens,[6] not in women as reproducers (WGNRR 1996c). Indian women in the health movement believe that the Cairo Conference converted women's health into an issue of safe abortion and reproductive rights; this conversion served to marginalize the issues of comprehensive primary health care, social security, and investments in other needed infrastructure like health facilities (WGNRR 1995). Indian women's groups wonder what purpose broadening the concept of maternal health to reproductive health serves when trained midwives (who represent the only professionalized medical care available in the countryside) conduct no more than 13 percent of rural home deliveries.

Another issue dividing women's groups is the emphasis on the individual in the rights discourse. Governments infringe on individuals' rights to marry and found a family (article 16 of the UN Universal Declaration of Human Rights) whenever they tie social welfare benefits to family size, and they create a conflict between what they say is the common good (slower rates of population growth) and individual reproductive choice. Some critics oppose the dichotomy between the individual and society as false: they point out that an emphasis on reproductive rights as individual demands rather than social rights fits neatly with neoliberal policies that make health an individual rather than a collective responsibility (The Corner House and WGNRR 2004).

To counter the narrow interpretation of reproductive rights as issues of choice and quality of care in conception, contraception, and birth control, many women's groups add sexuality. The Women's Health Project in South Africa suggests a sexual rights framework for men and women that embodies the right to have control over one's own body; have sex when, with whom, and how one wants and not be forced to have sex; make decisions about one's own sexuality; have sexual enjoyment; protect oneself from the risk of the consequences of sex, such as pregnancy, sexually transmitted infections, and AIDS; and have access to nonjudgmental, responsive services that help deal with sexual health concerns (Hlatshwayo and Klugman 2001).

Women's health advocates recognize that population policies will continue in the future making collaboration with feminists and sympathetic people in the establishment necessary to the transformation of population policies, contraceptive research, and family planning programs. Their aim is to ensure women's reproductive health and rights, efforts described in the rest of this chapter.

Population Dynamics

All societies have population regimes, managing family size through a variety of social controls and practices; historically these controls have included infanticide, birth spacing through prolonged breastfeeding and the imposition of taboos on sexual relations before the baby is weaned, and the use of herbal contraceptives and abortifacients (Cordell, Gregory, and Piché 1987). A bias against girls dominates current practices: selective abortion and infanticide to eliminate females, neglect of girls in favor of boys who have first claims to food and medical attention, and domestic violence against girls and women. The United Nations estimates that every year from 1.5 to 3 million women and girls lose their lives as a result of gender-based violence or neglect and from 113 to 200 million women around the world are demographically "missing" (Ali 2006). Societies with a strong preference for sons over daughters are using modern technologies to determine the sex of the fetus and to abort females. When daughters are born, parents frequently give them up for adoption, sometimes to families in another country.

Many state policies affect rates of population growth: war, peace, and diplomacy; laws regulating health and safety in homes and workplaces, and access to food and water as well as health care, housing, and jobs, all of which affect death rates; emigration and immigration policies; and systems controlling income, including taxes, education, and pensions, which distribute wealth and poverty. In view of this broad range of factors, population studies that focus almost exclusively on fertility, almost always on women, and usually on chemical and surgical controls of birth, seem curiously narrow. Even more simplistic is the neo-Malthusian view that zero population growth will solve social and economic problems, or put more gently, that excessive population is a major cause of poverty and that lowering fertility will facilitate prosperity (Hodgson and Watkins 1997). Contemporary Malthusian arguments are not just simplistic but impervious to rational criticism: evidence has small effect on discussions about how to deal with "overpopulation" (Lohmann 2003).

Wars, which set in train famines, exoduses, and spikes in death and disability, are primary determinants of population patterns. Yet the dynamics of population in war zones and in the aftermath of war are poorly studied aspects of demography; few assessments go beyond the enumeration of internally displaced persons and refugees (Taipale 2002). Wartime census bureaus usually do not collect health and population data, and conflicting estimates of mortality and morbidity are part of the propaganda of warring sides. As might be expected, war-related mortality is sex- and age-selective and specific, with higher deaths rates in three groups—adult men and young boys who are fighting, the elderly (usually disproportionately women), and children (see Turshen 2004 for more details). One obvious consequence of the higher mortality among adult men is more widows and more female-headed households in war-torn societies.

War creates a pronatalist environment, putting pressure on women, affecting their reproductive choices, and resulting in the phenomenon known after the Second World War as the postwar baby boom. Demographers have done almost no research on this phenomenon in the aftermath of other wars, although scattered observations suggest it might be widespread. A study of the Dinka in an emergency relief center in Southwestern Sudan, where war raged intermittently for 40 years, concluded that families desire many children to replace the infants lost to war (Jok 1999). But the recalcitrance of young Dinka women who agree to conceive only reluctantly thwarts family desires; as many as 35 percent terminate pregnancy, resorting to unsafe and clandestine abortion and risking infertility, infection, or death. In Palestine, where a foreign power has occupied the territory for over 40 years, an already high birth rate rose steeply during the first *intifada*, the nationalist uprising that began in 1987, reaching 46.7 and 54.7 per 1,000 in 1990 in the West Bank and the Gaza Strip, respectively (UN 2005). Although generally a matter of choice, not coercion, and women speak proudly of raising many children to help in the fight for independence, the impact of the soaring birth rate further exacerbates the inequality of men's and women's lives. In northeastern Uganda, where conflict with the Lord's Resistance Army has been going on since 1987, the population growth rate is 4.6 percent, compared with 3.2 percent for the country as a whole (Uganda Bureau of Statistics 2002). Research by ISIS-WICCE over six years reveals that, among other factors, the lack of family planning services in the region has left many women and girls with no protection against pregnancy (Ojiambo Ochieng 2003).

Birth Control and Contraception

Colonial legacies and the Catholic Church dominate the record of government regulation of birth control practice in the global South. The European powers imposed on their colonies—in the legislation they adopted to govern their subjects and in their parochial attitudes towards women and childbearing—their gender, race, and class prejudices as well as the labor force needs of their economies. In the late nineteenth and early twentieth centuries the racist eugenics movement (described below) advocated the use of sterilization and contraception for selected groups in Europe and the Americas. Eugenics made surgical contraceptive procedures performed by doctors acceptable. Birth control for the masses, however, was still restricted: in 1873 the U.S. Congress passed the Comstock Act, making birth control a federal crime, contraceptives obscene and illicit, and interstate sales of birth control devices illegal. Although in the twentieth century urbanization contributed to popular demands for reliable methods of birth control to cope with rising costs of childrearing, and women and men were demanding more individual control over their lives, and even though colonial armies needed better protection from venereal diseases, governments refused to legalize contraception. Great Britain continued to restrict access to contraception and abortion in the countries of its colonial empire long after the British women's movement achieved change at home in the 1930s.[7]

As Asian, Middle Eastern, and African countries liberated themselves from colonial rule in the decades after the Second World War, few new governments repealed those laws (and most still retain the ban on abortion). In the 1960s, warnings about a world "population explosion" coincided with Rockefeller Fund investment in research on women's fertility and the development of the contraceptive pill. Not until the population control establishment gathered momentum in the 1970s did contraception begin to become available, and then not as a routine aspect of gynecological care (as WHO recommended) but as part of vertical family planning campaigns. Women's health movements continue to fight the colonial legacy as well as the population control establishment.

Women's health movement veterans of the fights for birth control and contraception North and South sense that their struggles are never ending, that no achievement is secure, that the population control establishment has reneged on its promises, and that the rise of religious fundamentalisms threatens every gain. Indian women wonder why contraceptive efficacy is more desirable than contraceptive safety (WGNRR 1995). Filipinas ask why antiabortion groups like Abay Pamilya distort the truth and support the ban on the emergency contraceptive pill, claiming that it is an abortifacient (WGNRR 2002e). The Reproductive Health Advocacy Network points out that the pill works in one of three ways: by interrupting ovulation (by delaying or inhibiting it), by inhibiting fertilization (by altering tubal transport of sperm or ova), or by altering the endometrium (thereby inhibiting implantation of the egg). It is not an abortifacient.

The following sections discuss women's responses to sterilization and abortion, the most controversial of birth control methods—sterilization because of its permanence and frequently involuntary nature, and abortion because it terminates pregnancy and evokes questions about the beginning of life. Raging arguments over the ethics of both methods do not prevent their widespread use by women all over the world (Hartmann 1995).

Sterilization

Sterilization is the most prevalent form of contraception worldwide (about 20 percent of women and 3.5 percent of men [UNDESA 2003]), not all of it voluntary. As a method of birth control, sterilization has a long political history tied to racism. This section looks at four cases—the United States, India, Peru, and Roma women in Slovakia—and considers quinacrine sterilization, a nonsurgical form of sterilization that women's health movements are campaigning against.

From the end of the nineteenth century, Argentina and Brazil used sterilization to eliminate indigenous people, favoring the immigration of Europeans and a process known as the "whitening" of the gene pool. The eugenics movement advocated the use of sterilization in Europe and North America in the first decades of the twentieth century to promote white supremacy by controlling the gene pool. The United States exported the technique to Nazi Germany (Black 2003). Along with passing state laws to prohibit interracial marriage and permit "eugenic sterilization," the eugenics movement also pressured governments in the United States and Great Britain to imprison "genetically inferior" women for the duration of their childbearing years, in effect sterilizing them (Zedner 1995). American eugenicists provided a biological rationale for the Immigration Act of 1924, which discriminated against immigrants from Eastern and Southern Europe. In 1927 the U.S. Supreme Court upheld eugenics programs that existed in at least 33 states and by their end had sterilized an estimated 65,000 people (Elliston 2003). Eugenicists promoted the program to economic elites, civic leaders, and social scientists as not just a means to "improve the race" but also a way to shrink welfare roles and reduce the black population.

United States

Among the U.S. states with extensive eugenics programs were North Carolina, Virginia, and California. Between 1929 and 1974, the North Carolina state government eugenics board authorized the surgical sterilization of more than 7,600 "feebleminded," "moronic," "delinquent," or "promiscuous" women (and some 75 men). More than 2,000 were under the age of 18. "Tellingly, as the civil rights movement gathered steam in the 1960s, the sterilizations, which already disproportionately targeted African Americans, were increasingly meted out against young blacks" (Elliston 2003, 11). The Disabled Action Committee, a national advocacy group based in Fairfax, Virginia, pressed successfully for the North Carolina state legislature to be the first in the country to express profound regret for the program. To its apology, which included regrets from the Wake Forest School of Medicine for its involvement, North Carolina added the creation of a historical archive (Markel 2003). The Governor of Virginia apologized in 2002 for the forced sterilization of some 7,500 people from 1924 to 1979 under the banner of eugenics, selective human breeding, or social engineering (WGNRR 2002c). The governors of Oregon, South Carolina, and California followed suit in the next 12 months. The Disabled Action Committee even launched a campaign to urge President George W. Bush to apologize for the federal government's role (Ragged Edge Online 2003).

Federal funding for sterilization, including a major campaign mounted in Puerto Rico in the 1940s (Hartmann 1995), continued through the years that white middle class women were demonstrating for the legalization of abortion (note that sterilization laws were on the books till 1974 in North Carolina and 1979 in Virginia). The U.S. government promoted permanent methods of population control for poor women and women of color, even as it restricted the use of nonpermanent methods of fertility control. Women of color—in nationalist organizations like Black Power, Black Panthers, and the Young Lords Party and in feminist organizations like the Black Women's Liberation Committee, the Third World Women's Alliance, and the Black Women's Liberation Group of Mount Vernon (New York)—argued that legal abortion was not synonymous with reproductive freedom and that the right to bear children was as important to reproductive freedom as the legal right to terminate a pregnancy (Nelson 2003). For Dorothy Roberts (1997) the chief danger of racist birth control policies is the legitimation of an oppressive social structure. Proposals to solve social problems by curbing black reproduction make racial inequality appear to be the product of nature rather than power. By identifying procreation as the cause of black people's condition, they divert attention away from the political, social, and economic forces that maintain America's racial order. In the years immediately preceding the 1973 Supreme Court decision legalizing abortion, the New York group Redstockings turned abortion into an issue of women's autonomy; and three years later CARASA redefined abortion rights as including the need to guarantee reproductive autonomy to even the poorest women.[8]

African Americans and Latinos were not the only targets of federally funded sterilization programs. U.S. government agency personnel, including the Indian Health Service, targeted American Indians for family planning because of their high birth rate. The 1970 census revealed that the average Indian woman bore 3.79 children, whereas the median for all groups in the United States was 1.79 children. American Indians have some of the highest sterilization rates in the country. The Indian Health Service sterilized at least 25 percent of Native American women between the ages of 15 and 44 during the 1970s. American Indians allege that the Indian Health Service failed to provide women with necessary information regarding sterilization; used coercion to get signatures on the consent forms; used improper consent forms; and did not wait an appropriate 72 hours between the signing of a consent form and the surgical procedure (Lawrence 2000).

Choctaw-Cherokee physician Dr. Connie Pinkerton-Uri conducted a study in 1974 that revealed Indian women generally agreed to sterilization when they were threatened with the loss of their children or their welfare benefits, that most of them gave their consent when they were heavily sedated during a Cesarean section or when they were in a great deal of pain during labor, and that the women could not understand consent forms because they were written in English at the twelfth-grade level. Dr. Pinkerton-Uri does not believe the sterilizations occurred from any plan to exterminate American Indians, but rather from the warped thinking of doctors who believe the solution to poverty is not to allow people to be born (Lawrence 2000).

Just as this chapter of U.S. history was coming to a close, a reactionary organization called CRACK (Children Requiring a Caring Kommunity, now called Project Prevention) started a program to permanently or temporarily sterilize women with substance abuse problems. Touring U.S. cities, CRACK targets low-income neighborhoods offering women $200 to either accept sterilization or use a long-acting reversible contraceptive like Norplant (Caton 2002). When CRACK came to Albuquerque, New Mexico, Young Women United, a community-based organization committed to the health and safety of teenagers and young adult women of color, teamed up with the Religious Coalition for Reproductive Choice and local allies to oppose CRACK's program of coerced sterilization.

India

In the global South, the population control establishment seemed to overcome the historical link between sterilization and the discredited eugenics movements and use vasectomies and tubectomies as standard methods of birth control in family planning campaigns. The United States Agency for International Development (USAID) funds the international program budget of the Association for Voluntary Surgical Contraception, which was formerly linked with the eugenics movement; AVSC (now called EngenderHealth) works in over 60 countries including India.

In 1975 Indian Prime Minister Indira Gandhi declared a state of emergency and introduced a family planning scheme that consisted of mass sterilization campaigns aimed at families with two or more children. Vasectomy was the preferred operation but the campaign also performed tubal ligations; the government offered incentives of cash, promotions, and raises to employees who recruited "acceptors" and filled their quota; those who refused or failed faced dismissal (Tarlo 2000). In New Delhi, the main target was the unskilled labor force, and from 1976 family planning programs combined with slum clearance: acceptance meant resettlement on a plot of land, refusal meant demolition of one's home with no replacement. At its height in 1975–1976, the campaigns sterilized more than 8 million Indians, most of them men, killed 1,774, and contributed to the downfall of the government (Bandarage 1997). Although the new government eliminated direct forms of compulsion, female sterilization became a central strategy in the renamed Family Welfare Program. Conditions in tubectomy camps are often unsanitary and can cause death. Cases of health-care providers performing coercive sterilizations still occur.[9]

The National Population Policy adopted in 1995 reflects the Cairo consensus, but according to Rao (2005) the practice in states does not conform. In Andhra Pradesh, more than half of married women have had tubal ligations, one of the highest rates in the world, because of the state's aggressive promotion of sterilization (*New York Times* 22 June 2001). In Rajasthan, a state subject to frequent droughts, the local government linked food relief to family planning (despite a central government decision not to); sterilization was a condition for participation in food relief employment schemes, and health workers registered the names of women who did not comply. "Coercion reached a pitch when women were forcibly operated on for a second or third time." (Sawhney 1999, 170) A two-child norm joins this emphasis on sterilization, and at least six states have mandated a two-child norm for members of village councils; some are extending it to civil servants as well on the notion that they should provide models of restraint. The consequences are dramatic for beneficiaries of a 1992 constitutional amendment that reflects India's effort to broaden democracy: the law reserves one-third of council seats for women and a certain number of state positions for lower-caste citizens, according to their proportion in the population. The two-child norm is now unseating some of those who have gained access to power for the first time. In Chhattisgarh, with more than 20 million people, 40 percent of them below the poverty line, the two-child norm went into effect in January 2001. State officials could not provide figures on how many *panchayat* members have faced dismissal since then, but several districts reported more than 100 cases each (Waldman 2003).

Peru

The United Nations and international aid agencies hailed the Peruvian family planning campaign in the mid-nineties, which they supported despite the fact that it sterilized over 350,000 men and women against their will. President Alberto Fujimori, facing genocide charges, said his aim was to liberate men and women from the burden of poverty and large families. A government report about the scandal exposes a sinister military plan, called Plan Verde, to exterminate entire social groups such as the poor and criminals. Military and intelligence sources in the report are all anonymous, but according to one source, a former military officer, the military deployed to sterilize people. One of the doctors responsible for the sterilizations, Dr Washington, is unrepentant despite the evidence against him. "Many women are very happy for what was done to them. They have less children, definitely, but they are happy" (http://www.insightnewstv.com/d68/ accessed 28 June 2006).

Reports of forcible sterilization in remote rural areas of Peru began circulating in the Lima press in 1997. Two women reportedly died because of the hasty and unsanitary conditions in which health workers carried out the sterilization procedures. Many women complained that government bureaucrats pressured them to have tubal ligations with warnings that they would lose their food subsidies if they refused to submit to the procedure; others reported that hospitals promised to waive childbirth expenses if they agreed to sterilization. According to the Peruvian Medical Federation, the Ministry of Health offered monetary incentives to physicians based on the number of sterilizations performed, and some doctors feared losing their jobs if they did not meet their quota (Burt 1998).

Peruvian public health officials threatened María Mamerita Mestanza Chávez with criminal sanctions in 1996 if she did not undergo sterilization. Her husband ultimately agreed to the surgery. No doctor examined her prior to the operation and complications ensued. Public health workers refused her medical treatment; she died at home nine days later.

After domestic legal remedies failed, the Latin American and Caribbean Committee for the Defense of Women's Rights (CLADEM) and two other Peruvian human rights group filed a petition in 1999 with the Inter-American Commission on Human Rights. In 2002 the Peruvian government agreed in principle to settle the case. The following year the government signed an agreement acknowledging international legal responsibility, agreeing to compensate Mestanza's surviving husband and children. The government also said it would implement the recommendations of Peru's Human Rights Ombudsman concerning sterilization procedures in Peru's government facilities (Rousseau 2006).

Coercive sterilization in Peru illustrates the challenges and opportunities for women's movements working with governments and the dissension collaboration causes within the movement. The Manuela Ramos Movement (Manuela) administers the USAID-funded Reproductive Health in the Community Project. ReproSalud aims to bring innovative services to poor women, while also encouraging them to make more effective claims on government services. But these official links proved a disadvantage when the press circulated stories of government health service abuses. Manuela had to choose between quiet diplomacy and openly criticizing public services in ways that might play into the hands of right-wing forces that wanted to shut down all public reproductive health care (UNRISD 2000). Meanwhile the Movimiento Amplio de Mujeres (MAM) protested against the health ministry, calling for the health minister's resignation, and demanding broad access to all contraceptive methods, quality services, and free and informed consent. Manuela, the Flora Tristán Women's Center, and other women's organizations sitting on the Tripartite Working Group on the Follow-up to the Cairo Conference (an ad hoc consultative body on reproductive health composed of government representatives, NGOs, and international donor agencies), along with most opposition congresswomen, hesitated to condemn the regime forcefully for these abuses, partly because of the risk of losing all the gains made in family planning (Rousseau 2006). Only in 1999 did Mesa Tripartita issue a public statement acknowledging certain problems in the quality of the health services performed in some cases, and Manuela came out publicly against sterilization abuses. The health ministry eventually made changes that were favorable to women's rights (Garcia-Moreno and Claro 1994).

Roma Women

Roma women in Slovakia also say that doctors have sterilized them against their will, without their consent, or that they signed consent papers unwittingly—their illiteracy preventing them from reading the documents to which they affixed an "X" or thumbprint (Green 2003a). The Center for Reproductive Rights documented 110 sterilizations of young Roma women since 1989, as well as a pattern of forced Caesarean section deliveries and substandard care in segregated wards. Slovak doctors and government authorities denied all allegations and threatened to sue the authors of the report, *Body and Soul*, produced by the Centre for Civil and Human Rights (*Poradna pre obcianske a fudake preva*) and the Center for Reproductive Rights. The UN Special Rapporteur on the Right to Health complained about the problem in a letter sent jointly with two other UN special rapporteurs (on racism and on violence against women) to the Government of Slovakia (Commission on Human Rights 2005).

The government replied that the police had launched an investigation regarding the criminal offence of genocide. The UN special rapporteurs alleged that the police had not conducted the criminal investigation into the allegations concerning forced sterilization in an acceptable manner. The government invited the Faculty of Medicine at Comenius University in Bratislava to give their expert opinion on these issues. The expert team examined all the hospitals mentioned in the *Body and Soul* report, including the Gynaecology and Obstetrics Department of Krompachy Hospital. These parallel inspections of health care establishments, which extended to 67 gynecology and obstetrics departments in the republic, complemented the criminal investigation. The team did not establish that the health care establishments had committed genocide, segregation, or discriminatory practices. The examination had revealed certain shortcomings in Slovak health legislation and administrative omissions on the part of doctors and/or health establishments in connection with obtaining informed consent of patients. However, the government explained that staff always respected medical indications for sterilization. A new law drafted as part of an extensive health care reform in the Slovak Republic would eliminate the legislative shortcomings revealed during the investigation in the case of alleged forced sterilizations (Commission on Human Rights 2005).

Quinacrine Sterilization

Quinacrine is a drug first used to treat malaria in the 1920s; researchers developed other medical applications such as the treatment of giardiasis, a parasitic infection, and in the 1970s Chilean scientists created quinacrine pellets as a method of nonsurgical, irreversible, female sterilization (Hartmann 1995). Seven pellets of 36 mg. of quinacrine inserted into the top of the uterus cause inflammation and scarring; the scarred tissue permanently closes the fallopian tubes (Rao 1997). The insertions require no anesthesia, no surgical facilities, and no physicians. For these reasons and because quinacrine is in the public domain and researchers cannot patent it, quinacrine sterilization is less expensive than tubal ligation. Without a patent, pharmaceutical companies cannot expect great profits and therefore have not financed clinical trials (Bhattacharyya 2003). As a drug in the public domain, quinacrine's use for sterilization is legal off label (off-label use is the practice of prescribing drugs for a purpose outside the scope of the drug's approved label). The U.S.-based NGO, Center for Research on Population and Security, run by doctors E. Kessel and S.D. Mumford, with funding from groups opposed to immigration into the United States, supports quinacrine trials in Bangladesh, India, and Chile (Rao 1997).

The Quinacrine Alert Network, a multiracial alliance of feminists, health practitioners, and scholars, is campaigning against the use of quinacrine because it increases the risk of ectopic pregnancy, and uterine complications can lead to hysterectomy. The lack of studies to rule out adverse effects like birth defects, genetic mutations, and cancer has women's health activists worried (WGNRR 2002b; www.drwhitney. com accessed 10 April 2007). According to the Committee on Women, Population and Environment, even though the U.S. Federal Drug Administration has not approved the method, Family Planning, Inc., a private clinic in Daytona Beach, Florida, advertises and offers quinacrine sterilization (WGNRR 2002c). The greater concern is the potential for abuse in the global South.

The International Federation of Gynecology and Obstetrics (FIGO) devoted an entire supplement of its official publication to quinacrine sterilization in 2003 (*International Journal of Gynecology and Obstetrics* 83 Suppl. 2). The supplement included 25 articles from 14 countries and reported on 40,242 cases (fewer than one third of the 140,000 women who have used the method). In its editorial, FIGO concluded that the method is safe, effective, and attractive to and well tolerated by women: "earlier concerns about increased ectopic [pregnancy] rates and carcinogenicity have not been borne out by the data so far accumulated." The editors support their conclusion by citing the long-term clinical experience with quinacrine sterilization, especially the large numbers of users in Vietnam. Hartmann (1995) calls Vietnam's population program heavy-handed and notes allegations of coercive use of quinacrine there: in 1993 the Vietnamese publication *The Woman* exposed the case of 100 women on the Hoa Binh rubber plantation who had quinacrine insertions without their knowledge (they thought they were having routine checks for intrauterine devices).

Women's movements continue to protest against the use of nonsurgical sterilization. The All India Democratic Women's Association led the call that resulted in India's governmental ban on quinacrine sterilization. A related international campaign—to stop research on immunological contraceptives—has been mobilizing women since 1993. By 1996, 450 groups from all over the world had signed a petition to stop research on antifertility vaccines. Research on a vaccine started in the early 1970s to create antibodies in a long-lasting vaccine that users could self-administer. Once again the concern is the potential for abuse: unethical trials with uninformed, nonconsenting women, and research driven not by women's needs but by concern with rapid population growth. Women also worry about unacceptable medical risks: immunological birth control methods turn the immune system against human reproductive cells or hormones. Among the campaign's successes were the agreement of the International Development Research Center of Canada to stop funding the research in India and the establishment at the World Health Organization of a Gender Advisory Panel to give a gender perspective on the agency's contraceptive activities and research (WGNRR 2003a).

Abortion

Currently 38.8 percent of the world's inhabitants live in the 127 countries that completely prohibit abortion or allow it only to protect a woman's life or health; an estimated 20 million women have abortions in these countries each year (CRLP 2006; Sai 2004).[10] Restrictions and prohibitions resulting in unsafe abortions are responsible for between 34,000 and 70,000 deaths annually, about 13 percent of pregnancy-related deaths (Berer 2002; Grimes 2003). Many of the laws prohibiting abortion in the global South date from the colonial period; few governments repealed them on gaining independence.

The health rationale, which frames abortion as a major contributing factor to women's mortality, is one of the approaches women's health advocates developed as a strategy for legalizing abortion. In Thailand, most advocacy work to legalize abortion has concentrated on the health rationale, stressing the high rates of morbidity and unnecessary mortality from complications following illegal abortions as well as the high attendant economic costs to the health system (Whittaker 2003). In Cameroon abortion is legal only in cases of rape or if the woman's life is in danger. The Cameroonian association to fight violence against women (*Association de lutte contre les violences faites aux femmes*) adopted the same strategy, cooperating with a number of local organizations to study abortion. Cameroonians created the Committee of Reflection on Abortion in 2002 to reduce maternal morbidity and mortality by focusing on unsafe abortions; the Committee met with the South African Women's Health Project and the International Women's Health Coalition the same year (Beleoken 2003). Some countries like Nigeria are using the health approach to frame abortion as a public health issue because they fear resistance to demands for legalization from the women's movement itself. Nigeria is one of a number of countries in which abortion is illegal but legal action against doctors or patients is uncommon (WGNRR 1996c).

A second approach is the human rights rationale, which asserts that fundamental principles of human rights protect the right to terminate a pregnancy. Women's rights advocates have criticized the health approach because it tends to define abortion in epidemiological and public health terms rather than as an issue of women's rights that must take account of their desires and experiences.

Some women's groups take the position that decriminalization is a more realistic goal than legalization. The September 28 Campaign for the Decriminalization of Abortion in Latin America and the Caribbean, created during the Fifth Latin America and Caribbean Feminist Encounter in Argentina in 1990, coordinates action in support of abortion. Catholics for a Free Choice in Uruguay[11] served as the first regional coordinating headquarters, a position that rotates among participating organizations; from 1994 GIRE (the Information Group on Reproductive Choice based in Mexico City) coordinated the campaign, followed by CIDEM (Bolivia), the Rede Feminista de Saúde (Brazil), and the Centro de la Mujer Peruana Flora Tristán. The principal goals of the campaign are to raise consciousness on the issue of sexual and reproductive rights and to work for the decriminalization of abortion throughout the region by promoting debate, reflection, and exchange of experience.

Peruvian feminists, gathered in a thematic collective dealing with reproductive and sexual rights, spoke out against the Chamber of Deputies' attempt in 1987 to modify abortion legislation by increasing legal sanctions; instead they asked for the decriminalization of abortion in order to put an end to its clandestine character with the goal of obtaining free access to a variety of efficient and safe contraceptive methods within the health system. The collective waged a similar battle between 1990 and 1991 when the government established the Commission for the Revision of the Penal Code. Feminists decided by consensus to adopt a multifaceted position as their strategy: one group emphasized the legalization of abortion, others pressured for decriminalization of abortion performed for economic and social reasons or for pregnancies resulting from rape (Barrig 1999). In 2005 the United Nations Human Rights Committee (UNHRC) decided its first abortion case. Peruvian state officials forced 17 year-old KL to carry a fatally impaired fetus to term. The decision establishes that denying access to legal abortion violates women's most basic human rights. This is the first time an international human rights body has held a government accountable for failing to ensure access to legal abortion services (UNHCR 2005).

U.S. women's groups made a strategic decision to emphasize privacy in the campaign to legalize abortion, and the Supreme Court affirmed the principles of the right to privacy and the protection of a woman's life and health in their 1973 decision, *Roe v. Wade*, which struck down state laws that restricted abortion. The strategy held through two major challenges to *Roe v. Wade*: the 1992 Court decision, *Sternberg v. Carhart*, which confirmed the privacy principle even as it extended limits on abortion, and the 1995 decision, *Planned Parenthood of Southeastern Pa v. Casey*, in which the Court reaffirmed that the Due Process clause of the U.S. Constitution protects the substantive force of liberty. "The Casey decision again confirmed that our laws and tradition afford constitutional protection to personal decisions relating to marriage, procreation, contraception, family relationships, childrearing, and education." (*New York Times* 27 June 2003) Despite these precedents, Congress approved, and President Bush signed, the Partial-Birth Abortion Ban Act of 2003 that would outlaw many abortion procedures performed throughout the second trimester, long before fetal viability, in violation of a woman's right to choose (Chavkin 2003). The law is part of an effort to hollow out the *Roe* decision that began almost as soon as the Court handed it down: the Hyde Amendment of 1977 (an amendment to Title XIX of the Social Security Act) prohibits the use of federal funds for abortion, effectively restricting access to abortion for low-income women. Some women's groups now question the strategy and argue that human rights of women would provide more invincible legal grounds than privacy.

From the beginning of the struggle to legalize abortion, women's groups have cooperated across borders: Irish women went to England, French women went to Switzerland, and U.S. women went from states with total restrictions to states with liberalized laws. Women on Waves is a Dutch NGO concerned to prevent unwanted pregnancy and unsafe abortions throughout the world (www.womenonwaves.org accessed 1 April 2007). Cooperating with local organizations, Women on Waves loads its mobile gynecological unit onto a ship and sails to countries to provide free reproductive health services including abortion (if necessary anchoring offshore to avoid the penalty where abortion is illegal). The ship sailed to Ireland in June 2001 and to Poland in June 2003 at the invitation of the Polish Federation for Women and Family Planning in Warsaw (Green 2003b). The plan was to offer free, early-term, medical abortions in international waters using the drug RU-486. Abortion is no longer legal in Poland; exceptions are rape, danger to the mother's life, or if the fetus has grave genetic defects.

Another example of women's transnational cooperation is the comparative study of advocacy for abortion access undertaken by the South African Women's Health Project (2001).[12] Working with NGOs advocating for abortion access North and South, the project provided 11 case studies of experiences for improving abortion access through legal change or by increasing access to and quality of services.

At the international level, until the administration of George W. Bush came to power in 2001 and imposed its restrictive vision of population control, family planning programs gradually included access to abortion in the declarations of international meetings. At the 1968 UN conference in Tehran, convened to assess progress made since the adoption of the 1948 Universal Declaration of Human Rights, governments agreed that parents have a basic right to determine freely and responsibly the number and spacing of their children. The 1974 World Population Conference in Bucharest expanded this consensus, acknowledging the right to information, education, and services to prevent unwanted pregnancy and ensure safe motherhood. The 1994 International Conference on Population and Development (ICPD), held in Cairo, stated: "In circumstances where abortion is not against the law, such abortion should be safe. In all cases women should have access to quality services for the management of complications arising from abortion." The Fourth World Conference on Women, held in Beijing the following year, stated that women should not be criminalized for having an abortion and that governments should consider reviewing laws containing punitive measures against women who have undergone illegal abortions.

Fetal Sex Selection

Gender bias influences the demand for abortion—a rejection of daughters that is more than a preference for sons. Medical authorities justify fetal sex selection on genetic grounds, since the X- and Y-chromosomes carry some hereditary diseases. In some instances fetal sex selection is benign; for example, couples with a boy may want a girl to achieve the "perfect balance." Microsort, based in Fairfax, Virginia, at the Genetics & IVF Institute, advertises sperm separation to prevent X-linked diseases and for family balancing (www.microsort.net accessed 1 April 2007). A Belgian fertility center in Ghent offers Microsort's sperm-sorting service to enable couples to select the sex of their next child. Microsort separates frozen sperm bearing Y-chromosomes from those carrying X-chromosomes and sends the sorted sperm back to Belgium for implantation (WGNRR 2003d). The Canadian government penalizes 13 practices related to reproduction, including sperm sorting, illustrating the trend to outlaw such practices for nonmedical purposes. The Canadian Human Reproductive and Genetic Technologies Act of 1996 penalizes prenatal sex selection for nonmedical reasons and any failure to obtain informed consent for the use of donated eggs, sperm, or embryos; the penalties include long maximum prison sentences (WGNRR 1996b).

In China and India the desire for sons or rejection of daughters drives the use of prenatal scans and the decision to abort female fetuses. Prenatal sex identification techniques, such as the ultrasound-B, represent a change from infanticide and abandonment of female children, widely practiced in China before 1950; put another way, they represent a change from female disadvantage in mortality to female disadvantage in natality (Bossen 2005). The result of so many aborted female fetuses is imbalanced sex ratios: since the 1980s, the sex ratio at birth has risen significantly in China with more than 121 boys for every 100 girls born in 1993 and 1994, and the 2000 census confirms this trend. In India the M/F birth ratio was 111 to 100 during the period 1996 to 1998. The normal ratio at birth is around 106, and worldwide the sex ratio is an estimated 101, meaning that there are 101 men for every 100 women. Sex selection reflects women's low social status and reinforces it.

In societies where son preference is strong, fetal sex selection threatens to disrupt society, but just how is a matter of controversy and debate. Chinese analysts say the inability of young men to find wives results not only in marriage pressure on young men, but also a series of social problems, such as inferior physical and psychological health of the unmarried, instability of marriages and families, births out of wedlock, lack of old age support for those who never married, increasing prostitution, and abduction of and trafficking in women (Jiang, Feldman, and Jin 2005). Some say a society with a relatively high proportion of young men is much more prone to violence, a sociobiological explanation that relies on crude evolutionary models of male behavior; others with an instrumental view of women's equality say it will impede the development of democracy and prosperity. No one can make accurate predictions about the effects because birth ratios began to skew only in 1985, when sex-selection technology spread; the extra boys born in the late 1980s are just now reaching adulthood (Glenn 2004).

Indian women campaigned for decades against the use of amniocentesis to determine the sex of the fetus, a campaign that led to passage of the Pre-Natal Diagnostic Techniques Regulation and Prevention of Misuse Act in 1994. The government banned misuse of medical techniques for fetal sex determination in the public health sector in the mid-1970s, and many states enacted legislation banning sex selection procedures. The State of Maharashtra, where the movement was strongest, was the first state in India to enact legislation in 1988; women's groups also demanded action from the Maharashtra Medical Council. Despite these laws, precedents, and attendant public discussion, medical malpractice is rampant and medical bodies fail to detect and punish guilty doctors. Women found it necessary in 1998 to form a coalition called the Tamil Nadu Campaign against Sex Selective Abortion (WGNRR 2001). On 4 May 2001, the Supreme Court of India took the government and other bodies to task for failing to implement the law. The judges commented,

> Unfortunately, developed medical science is misused to get rid of a girl child before birth. Knowing full well that it is immoral and unethical as well as it may amount to an offence, the foetus of a girl child is aborted by qualified and unqualified doctors or compounders. This has affected the overall sex ratio in various states where female infanticide is prevailing without any hindrance. (Jesani, Madwidalla, and Gupte 2001, 16)

Why are the solutions proposed so ineffective? One answer is that the doctors who perform sex selective abortions believe they are providing an important social service; another is that antinatal groups believe these abortions will control population growth (Kishwar 2002). Third, Indian women's groups face a dilemma over fetal sex selection and reproductive choice: as more and more women use the right to abortion for selective abortion of female fetuses, Indian women's groups ask how the movement can advocate for abortion rights while contesting population policies and sex selection at the same time. Fourth, sex selective abortion reflects the spread of upper caste and upper class preferences to lower status groups and the customs of the northern and western regions of the country to the south and east (Kishwar 2002). Finally, the most significant reason for popular resistance to the ban is probably the increasing shortage of land, which pushes peasant families to have sons who will work the land and keep it in the family. Nonetheless, the government is committed to enforcing laws designed to curb fetal sex selection, and in March 2006 the courts found guilty and jailed for two years a doctor who revealed the sex of a female fetus and then agreed to abort it (Huggler 2006).

Infertility

Among the early demands of women from the South in redefining the abortion movement as reproductive rights in the 1980s was the addition of treatment for infertility. Women's groups in the global North and South made this demand at the International Conference on Population and Development held in Cairo in 1994. Rising rates of infertility have spawned new technologies, bringing benefits and disappointments as well as abuses, but no research on causes or prevention. The World Health Organization (WHO 2003) defines infertility as the inability to conceive within 12 months (within six months for a woman 35 years or older) or to carry a pregnancy to live birth. WHO estimates that infertility affects over 80 million people in the world today, most of them in developing countries. In the worst affected areas of the South, over 30 percent of couples may be infertile, mainly because of damage to the woman's reproductive tract caused by treatable infections like gonorrhea and chlamydia (WHO 2003). Despite the common perception that population growth rates are high throughout sub-Saharan Africa, infertility is common, reaching 30 to 40 percent in certain regions; infertility is a cause of divorce and an incentive for polygamy (Sow and Bop 2004). Common reasons for infertility in the North are later age at first marriage and starting a family later in life. Male infertility contributes to perhaps half of all cases worldwide, yet everywhere societies believe that infertility is a woman's problem (Inhorn 2003).

Finding it more difficult to conceive, couples are seeking help from specialists who use drug therapy or surgical procedures to treat them (Tarkan 2002). These treatments may not be successful, and about 5 percent of couples not helped go on to seek access to new reproductive techniques; where governments are not responsive, private services are meeting the need. By the mid-1990s, fertility clinics were treating 200,000 to 300,000 people in the United States; by 2001 over 100,000 had attempted in vitro fertilization (IVF is the technique of extracting eggs to fertilize them with sperm in the laboratory and implanting the embryo in the uterus), at charges of $12,500 to $25,000 with the woman's own eggs and $20,000 to $35,000 with donor eggs (Kolata 2004a). In 2001, 107,587 IVF attempts resulted in 21,813 live births (Kolata 2004a). Infertility treatment is a small segment of the profitable $10 billion market for women's pharmaceuticals, and in the 1990s the market for infertility drugs was growing at over 16 percent per year (Key and Marble 1996).

WHO (2003) has questioned the provision of these technologies in developing countries, given the expense and a success rate of less than 30 percent. For women in the global South, clearing up untreated gynecological problems like sexually transmitted infections is often sufficient for conception to occur. Because public hospitals generally do not provide assisted reproductive technologies, the poor have no access to these services. In Latin America, this discrimination has caused resentment.

Assisted reproductive technologies raise issues that are social, political, religious, and ethical as well as economic and financial. The technology promises liberation and enhanced human freedom but more often promotes conformity and reinforces the status quo (Roberts 1997). In India more than 60 centers offer assisted reproductive technologies, with no monitoring or regulation and little discussion of the moral, ethical, and social issues the technologies raise (WHO 2003). The government of Singapore responded to its country's falling birthrate by investing in the rapid development of new reproductive technologies, including the world's first egg bank and micro-insemination sperm transplant (a technique used to increase sperm count); Singapore directed these services to the educated elite Chinese population, not the Indians or the majority Malays (Roberts 1997). In the United States these technologies carry a racist subtext: the users are almost exclusively whites with the money to preserve genetic ties between parents and children. Roberts (1997) believes the implicit message is that white people deserve to procreate while black people do not, potentially worsening racial inequality.

Providers of in vitro fertilization and artificial insemination currently operate in a legal and ethical vacuum, with virtually no state regulation (WHO 2003). Some of the controversies surrounding IVF are the definition of parenthood (Gabriel 1996), the legitimacy of children conceived in this way (Inhorn 2003), whether the biological mother should take more responsibility for her child's life, or, indeed, whether the biological mother has any rights over the child. Almost no research measures the impact of violations of women's reproductive rights—whether it is the use of interventionist practices (some of which have no scientific justification), denial of patient privacy, or failure to gain meaningful informed consent. In the section on the commodification of body parts we discuss questions revolving around incentives for donating eggs and for surrogacy.

Commodification of Body Parts

In response to the demand for body materials, more and more people are selling parts of themselves—of concern here is the sale of reproductive components (eggs, sperm, and fetal material) and the "rental" of wombs—usually because of their poor economic circumstances. The high-tech entrepreneurs who broker these sales are reaping billions of dollars in profit. These practices make women and men witting and unwitting manufacturers of new commodities, including for their own use, and enable the wealthy to buy the genetic material of the poor.

Sperm is the leading reproductive commodity currently on sale: about 172,000 women per year in the United States use sperm in artificial insemination, a procedure with a 38 percent success rate. Companies pay sperm "donors" about $50 per transaction. The second procedure in the infertility marketplace is the harvest of eggs; unlike sperm ejaculation, egg donation is a risky medical procedure. Egg harvesting is invasive and incurs grave risks of hemorrhage, infection, cancer, and infertility.[13] In the United States fertility clinics "compensate" young women who "donate" their eggs (Lerner 1996); the going rate is currently $8,000. The high cost has given rise to a trade in human ova: Romanian women "earn" about $270 per donation (BBC News 23 December 2004); South Africa, with its rich racial heritage (and high levels of poverty), "pays" donors $500 (*Le Figaro* 31 March 2005).

Aborted fetuses are used in research or in transplants; harvesting fetal tissue and fetal parts—the supply in the United States is estimated at 1.6 million per year and in the world at 30 million—requires substantial alterations in the method, timing, and manner of abortions because fetal tissue is effective only if it is reasonably developed (usually second trimester), intact, and alive (Kimbrell 1993). The International Institute for the Advancement of Medicine (a U.S.-based, private, not-for-profit company) pays a "service fee" to abortion clinics that perform second-trimester abortions to supply its specialists with fetuses from which they extract fetal parts for researchers, charging a fee of between $50 and $150 per specimen.

Surrogate motherhood entails a couple paying a woman to gestate their baby, using the man's sperm and the woman's own egg, a donated egg, or the egg of the surrogate. Surrogate motherhood arrangements, colloquially described as the rental of wombs, value a man's capacity to be a genetic father over a mother's biological relationship to the child. Surrogacy raises class issues when poor women carry the children of wealthy couples, a contract complicated by racial issues when couples from the North turn to women in the South. As with egg donors, surrogates may consent to the procedure without adequate knowledge of their legal rights or the ability to hire a lawyer should the need arise. Surrogacy is a profitable business, with baby brokers negotiating commercial contracts.

The first case of surrogate motherhood in India in 1997 brought out the need for clear ethical guidelines, which the Indian Council of Medical Research (ICMR) developed but which the government has not yet implemented (WHO 2003). Surrogate mothers in India are a bargain for foreigners. Payment usually ranges from about $2,800 to $5,600, and the cost of the in vitro fertilization and surrogacy process totals about $7,200 (Chu 2006). Even with travel expenses factored in, the overall cost works out to much less than in the United States, where surrogacy costs a minimum of $35,000 to $40,000.[14] Some Indians like S.K. Nanda, a former health secretary in Gujarat state, see the practice as a logical outgrowth of India's fast-paced economic growth and liberalization of the last 15 years, a perfect meeting of supply and demand in a globalized marketplace. "It's win-win . . . a completely capitalistic enterprise. There is nothing unethical about it. If you launched it somewhere like West Bengal or Assam [both poverty-stricken states] you'd have a lot of takers." (Quoted in Chu 2006) The ICMR estimates that helping residents and visitors beget children could bloom into a nearly $6-billion-a-year industry. India has no laws regulating the fertility industry, only the ICMR's nonbinding guidelines.

U.S. courts have ruled both ways in cases in which surrogates have wanted to keep the baby after birth, sometimes awarding the child to the birth mother and sometimes to the contracting couple. In the latter cases, the courts variously call the birth mother the gestational carrier of the child, a host, a maternal environment, or fetal environment (Kimbrell 1993).

Like the debates in India over fetal sex selection and women's right to choose, women's health movements are divided over the issue of surrogacy: is it a woman's decision or should it be regulated by more than contract law?

Breasts and Other Body Parts

One of the more curious trends in the commercialization of body parts is the commodification of women's breasts through surgical implants, as well as the $4.6 billion brassiere market, which offers inflatable brassieres, padded brassieres, silicon gel and liquid inserts (Ferguson 2001). Breasts have symbolic meaning in many cultures, and attitudes toward breasts illustrate the social construction of women's health. In North America and Europe breasts are sex symbols used to sell unrelated products like automobiles. Breast implants originated in Japan after the Second World War where Japanese sex workers seeking to attract American occupying troops experimented with breast enlargement. With increasing rates of breast cancer in the North, physicians began to recommend implants following mastectomy (breast removal, the standard treatment for more than 60 years); this is the same surgery offered to women who for professional or personal reasons want larger breasts. Playing upon women's fear that they are no longer women when they have lost a breast to cancer, health workers urge breast implants or prostheses, telling women that prostheses are "better for the body" and "better than nothing." Breast "augmentation" is now the third most common cosmetic surgery in the United States with 291,000 operations performed in 2005 (www.fda.gov accessed 8 August 2006).

Women's groups have weighed the many pros and cons of implants marketed as beauty aids and concluded that silicone breast implants produce risks that outweigh the benefits to women. Some women take a less drastic position than an outright ban, suggesting that surgeons should give implants only when medically necessary, as after mastectomy; they also ask how to regulate surgeons who offer breast implants. Under pressure from women's groups and the U.S. Food and Drug Administration (FDA), manufacturers pulled silicone implants from the market in 1992. FDA reversed its decision again in 2006. Saline implants are available, but women who want implants for breast reconstruction after surgery for cancer or who simply want larger breasts say that silicone implants look and feel more natural.

Inamed (part of the Allergan corporation) based in Santa Barbara, California, applied to FDA for approval to return silicone implants to the market. The National Organization of Women (NOW), the National Women's Health Network, and Public Citizen's Health Research Group petitioned FDA to delay its review, citing entreaties from women who said that silicone implants had made them ill and ruined their lives. Hundreds of thousands of women have claimed that implants caused cancer, autoimmune and neurological diseases, and chronic fatigue syndrome. In mid-October 2003, FDA's panel of experts recommended approval of the return of silicone implants to the market, citing lack of conclusive scientific evidence linking implants to serious disease.[15] The panel confirmed this ruling in 2006.

Body Modification or Body Mutilation

Breast implants are one of many procedures that permanently alter appearance. With no common definition of beauty and sexuality in women, the temporary and permanent ways women enhance their beauty differ widely from one culture and context to another. What appears to be beautification in one may seem like mutilation and violation of the human right to bodily integrity in another. To explore how culturally bound and contextualized such procedures are, it is useful to try to classify them and ask what criteria one uses to categorize customs and procedures as body modification or body mutilation.

Is there a difference between breast implants after mastectomy and implants in exotic dancers who want to enhance their appearance? Is there a difference between implants for medically diagnosed micromastia (colloquially, flat-chested women) and for a male-to-female sex change? What about breast removal as prophylaxis against genetically inherited breast cancer and breast reduction for women or men (diagnosed with gynecomastia), or for a female-to-male sex change?

Many women react with revulsion to genital cutting and call it female genital mutilation; but what about surgical correction of ambiguous genitalia, correction of an enlarged clitoris, and laser rejuvenation of the vagina? Male circumcision is a religious ritual (not equivalent to female genital cutting); some criticize the rite as no better than castration to create eunuchs. But what about castration for male-to-female sex change? Another custom that attracts feminist study is foot binding in China: is it like breast binding, wearing girdles and bras, or even stiletto heels and tight jeans that deform the body?

Since Emancipation, people consider the branding of slaves a form of body mutilation and the tattooing of prisoners a Nazi war crime but, in the context of current fashion, tattoos, scarification, and body piercing are merely modifications. What changes our perceptions? Why is limb amputation to create better beggars unacceptable, but limb amputation for diabetics acceptable, and why is amputation as punishment controversial? What about limb extension, an operation popular among people who want to be taller? Is the use of growth hormones to increase height more acceptable than surgery?

Cosmetic surgery is now a hugely profitable industry, but should surgical repair of malformations like cleft palate and stomach stapling to reduce obesity be lumped in with facelifts, nose jobs, surgical body sculpting, and liposuction? How do we distinguish between the forced feeding of hunger strikers and the traditional fattening brides in Polynesia? How do medical doctors justify their participation in torture to extract information from prisoners?

Some criteria for deciding whether a procedure is modification or mutilation of the body are: is it voluntary or coerced? If voluntary, at what age does one elect the procedure and what constitutes consent? Is the purpose a medical necessity or is the procedure elective? But these questions raise further ones: what is voluntary in the context of cultural norms and peer pressure? Who defines purpose, especially of medical procedures? A movement of people born with ambiguous genitalia protests surgical correction of the condition (Intersex Society of North America www.isna.org/FAQ.html accessed 8 August 2006). What about age when, according to surgeons, many operations are more successful if performed in childhood? Labeling a custom body modification or body mutilation is difficult because such procedures are culturally determined and contextually circumscribed. Which rites are really human rights violations, infringing on bodily integrity?

Breast Cancer and Cervical Cancer

Given the obsession with breast size in many cultures, it seems paradoxical that the medical profession paid so little attention to breast cancer, one of the two most important cancers for women (the other is cancer of the cervix). In the global South, cervical cancer is the more common of the two (20 percent of new cancers), particularly among women who have little access to routine gynecological care, have given birth to many children, had many sexual partners, or whose partners were promiscuous (Paolisso and Leslie 1995). Breast cancer is more common among women in higher income countries exposed to a polluted environment who have had fewer or no pregnancies (Epstein 1994).

Cervical cancer and breast cancer illustrate, in different ways, how women's health movements have changed health research, medical practice, and health service delivery. When South African women started the Women's Health Project in the early 1990s, they consulted widely with NGOs, women's groups, church groups, political organizations, and trade unions, asking them about their priorities. The groups repeatedly mentioned cervical cancer so the Women's Health Project developed a policy proposal that thousands of South African women reviewed. The revised proposal—to screen women over 30 years of age three times in their life and to focus first on screening every woman who has never had a pap smear—then went to the new government for implementation; with government approval the Women's Health Project began to work with clinics, laboratories, and hospitals to help build the system that could deliver cervical screening (Fonn 2004).

In contrast to the South African inexpensive public health approach to cervical cancer, the United States is considering making compulsory for 11 to 12 year-old girls an expensive vaccine. Promoted by Merck pharmaceuticals, the vaccine producer, the program entails a series of three shots over a period of six months at a cost of $360 (http://www.kaiseredu.org/topics_im.asp?parentID=72&imID=1&id=609 accessed 12 April 2007). Effectiveness beyond five years and the long-term consequences are unknown, and because the vaccine does not protect against all kinds of HPV (human papilloma virus, which causes cervical cancer), pap smears will still be needed.

Changes in the treatment of breast cancer began with the work of one woman patient, Rose Kushner; in 1975 she wrote, *Breast cancer: a personal history and investigative report*, challenging the practice of radical mastectomy, the only treatment available, and the medical profession's "refusal to grant any measure of autonomy or even choice to the women whose malignancies they were treating in such routine and standardized fashion" (Kushner 1975, 53). By 1980 she had changed the mind of the cancer establishment, which began to make more options available to women. The movement she started urged scientists to undertake the research on which they eventually based lumpectomy and other modified operations.

Progress on prevention is slower, hampered by corporate interests and the nonprofit cancer societies they dominate. The pioneering epidemiologist Samuel Epstein disclosed the close ties between cancer organizations and big business such as oil and chemical companies as one reason researchers have not done better work on possible carcinogens, and why the national agenda for breast cancer research neglects environmental questions. Together with dissidents like Epstein, women's health movements began questioning the causes of breast cancer and geographical and racial variations in incidence and outcome. The response of the cancer establishment was predictable: instead of focusing on the 80 percent of cancers that are environmental in origin, scientists studied the perhaps 5 to 10 percent of breast cancer patients whose disease is due to mutations in the BRCA genes. When the black women's health movement in the United States pointed out that the incidence of breast cancer was lower in their community than among whites but that the death rate was higher, researchers responded with myriad studies of black "health care-seeking behavior," in effect blaming the victims for "bad" diets and late diagnoses that they said were the "causes" of higher mortality. Researchers mentioned the possibility of racial bias less frequently (Geiger 2002). When women asked for research on prevention, the cancer establishment launched large-scale studies of drugs like tamoxifen and raloxifene; healthy women surprised them, balking at the prospect of taking a drug for the rest of their lives to prevent a disease they might never develop. AstraZeneca, the sole manufacturer of tamoxifen, the world's top-selling cancer drug widely used for treating breast cancer, was behind the ill-advised National Cancer Institute trials to see whether tamoxifen can prevent the disease in healthy women, despite risks of complications that included uterine cancer, liver cancer, liver failure, blood clots, and crippling menopausal symptoms (Epstein and Rennie 1992).

Companies have been quick to take advantage of women's fears of breast cancer, launching marathons like Walk for Breast Cancer and Bicycle for Breast Cancer and sponsoring other fundraising efforts for research to fight breast cancer, which raise little money for research but provide great publicity for the companies. Breast cancer awareness month, which falls in October, has been an annual event in the United States since 1984. Conceived of by Imperial Chemical Industries, one of the world's largest petrochemical manufacturers, and its U.S. subsidiary and spin-off Zeneca Pharmaceuticals (now AstraZeneca), the American Cancer Society, the National Cancer Institute (NCI), the American College of Radiology, and mainstream women's groups enthusiastically promote the month (Epstein 1997). Powerful manufacturers of mammography equipment and film are behind this recommendation, despite international studies showing that routine premenopausal mammography is associated with increased breast cancer death rates at older ages and an annual cost in the United States of $2.5 billion (Epstein 1997). Major cosmetic companies—Avon, Revlon, Estée Lauder—market "pink ribbon" products during breast cancer awareness month. Breast Cancer Action, a group based in San Francisco, accuses the companies of hypocrisy, since dozens of their products contain toxic ingredients with possible links to breast cancer (*New York Times* 24 October 2003). For example, parabens, used as preservatives, are endocrine disruptors that mimic the hormone estrogen, and increased estrogen exposure over a lifetime is a proven risk factor for breast cancer. Phthalates help lotions penetrate the skin and make nail polish more flexible; phased out of baby toys because of its association with birth defects and developmental disabilities, phthalates are also endocrine disruptors.

U.S. women's health movements, following the path-breaking work of Barbara Seaman (1969), had to push the FDA to regulate the hormones in contraceptive pills, lowering the high dosages that were promoting breast cancer (see chapter 4 for a detailed discussion). Assisted by the work of the Health Research Group, women's health groups also pushed for regulation of mammography equipment that was emitting carcinogens, causing the very cancers they were designed to detect. Until the women's health movement won the victory of more government-funded research on women's health (the Women's Health Initiative), no large-scale studies could confirm the efficacy of annual mammograms or establish the age at which women should first start to have them. The consortium promoting Breast Cancer Awareness Month claims that since no prevention is available women should have regular mammograms for early detection, and they focus on women in the 40–50 age group.

Now with European researchers exposing the links between the American Cancer Society (and its British counterpart, the Royal Cancer Society) and the drug and mammography equipment makers, and between this industry and the conduct of large-scale surveys, everything in this field is up in the air. These researchers find no benefit from breast self-examination, mammograms before age 50, or mammograms more frequent than every two years for women over 50, and no long-term survival benefit of radical mastectomy over lumpectomy.

A coda to this story: at the end of 2006 researchers reported a precipitous drop in breast cancer rates in the United States. After increasing for almost seven decades, the rate fell in 2003, by 7 percent in the incidence of newly diagnosed breast cancers and by 15 percent among women with estrogen-fueled cancers. Scientists explained the drop by pointing to the corresponding decrease in the use of hormones for menopause that women abandoned when the Women's Health Initiative, the research program that the women's health movement had pressed the government to adopt, concluded that hormone therapy for menopause increased the risk of breast cancer. Dr V. Craig Jordan, vice president and scientific director for the medical science division at Fox Chase Cancer Center in Philadelphia said he was not surprised because, "we've known there is a cause and effect with hormones and breast cancer since 1896" (quoted in Kolata 2006).

CHAPTER SEVEN

Toward a New Universalism

In this final chapter we return to the discussion of the intersection of gender, race, and class (begun in chapter 2) in order to explore inequality in relation to difference, adding two more dimensions—disability and mental illness. My purpose is to disengage concepts of cultural difference from theories of economic difference, in order to consider class politics separately from ideas of identity politics. Movement activists have partially succeeded in moving definitions of women's health out of the biomedical sphere into a wider social framework, shifting the paradigm from biology to social relations. They have made less progress incorporating economic difference in social dynamics. Disability and mental illness, two areas in which medicine and biology strongly resist new social paradigms, are ideal subjects for an exploration of gender and class politics. The chapter concludes the discussion of difference and diversity with some thoughts about universalism and equality.

Disability

People living with disabilities—10 percent of the world's population—are among the poorest of the poor and frequently live on the margins of society. The three conceptual models of disability are the medical model, the social model, and the biopsychosocial model. The medical model views disability as a personal feature caused by disease, trauma, or other health condition, requiring medical care to correct the problem. It makes a pathology of difference and individualizes disability. The social model sees disability as a socially created problem, not as an attribute of an individual, demanding a political response; because an unaccommodating physical environment creates the problem, only a political response can change attitudes and other features of the social environment. The biopsychosocial model synthesizes what is "true in the medical and social models, without making the mistake each makes in reducing the whole, complex notion of disability to one of its aspects" (WHO 2002b). For WHO, the biopsychosocial synthesis, which is the basis of *The International Classification of Functioning, Disability and Health*, known commonly as ICF, provides a coherent view of different perspectives of health: biological, individual, and social.

Too many people perceive disability and the disabled person's lack of success as a personal problem stemming from an individual's medical impairment. But structural and attitudinal barriers are beyond an individual's control and these factors can turn a disability into a handicap. Economic inequality and prejudices surrounding age, race, ethnicity, gender, and class compound the discrimination that disabled people face. The systematic lack of access to education and employment, the failure of educational institutions and employers to make materials available in alternative formats for the visually and hearing impaired, barriers to wheelchair access to public services, and the bureaucracy that itself is a barrier to essential medical services and income supports are some of the structural factors that turn disability into handicap (Malhotra 2001). Sexism and racism are critical in turning a mild disability into a severe handicap.

Disability and Poverty

In the social environment model, features of the world—both natural and those human beings build and design—play a prominent role in the creation of the disadvantages that disabled people experience (Bickenbach et al. 1999). People with disabilities experience their impairments as a collection of socially created limitations that are discriminatory because they restrict opportunity for full and equal participation. Some social activists and advocates for persons with disabilities argue that disablement is a political issue, because persons with disabilities constitute a minority that society systematically discriminates against. The limitations the disabled face in education, employment, housing, and transportation are not the products of their medical condition but of social attitudes of neglect and stereotypical images of their capacities and needs. The minority group analysis was an outgrowth of scholarship and political activism rooted in popular political movements such as civil rights, consumer rights, independent living, deinstitutionalization, normalization, and antiprofessionalism. Note that the analysis did not arise from class politics or unionism. The unspoken question here is who provides and who pays for special education, the adaptation of workplaces and housing, and the transformation of public transit systems.

Another group insists that disablement is a universal human phenomenon that society systematically ignores with dire and unjust social consequences. The eminent sociologist Irving Kenneth Zola (1989), himself a polio survivor, argues that we need to recognize that the entire population is at risk for the concomitants of chronic illness and disability, that disability is an infinitely various but universal feature of the human condition. We need a political strategy that demystifies the specialness of disability. If we persist in seeing people with a disability as different with special needs, wants, and rights in a world of finite resources, then we are bound to pit them against the rest of the population. A useful analogy here is to debates about occupational health regulations—do we protect the individual woman working in a hazardous workplace that can affect her reproductive health or do we transform the workplace so that it is safe for all workers, male and female?

Zola's argument begins to move the debates out of the realms of biology and personal characteristics into society and class politics. The next step is to introduce the direct relationship between poverty and disability, which Sussman (1969) showed in his examination of U.S. data. Poverty is often a cause of disability when it is a barrier to good nutrition and good and timely health care, especially during pregnancy and childbirth. Poverty exposes girls and women to harmful or dangerous home, community, and workplace environments that may affect their development or that of a fetus (just as toxic chemical work environments can affect men, damaging the chromosomes in sperm). Poverty also increases the disadvantage of disabled people complicating their efforts to seek timely medical care, obtain education and training, or access enabling technology; good medical care, training, and technology could increase their likelihood of finding employment. The lack of all three makes the problem circular: disability can cause poverty.

Many disabled women in the South are more handicapped than their sisters with the same condition in the North. Because of poverty and sexism and because all kinds of resources are limited, women in the South are more handicapped than their condition suggests. Societal prejudices that diminish the status of disabled women can be more debilitating than the actual disability. The media portray disabled women as weak and vulnerable, and this image acts to perpetuate the negative public perception of the disabled. This difference between disability and handicap is in part due to general levels of development; high levels of development mean a public infrastructure that increases access (for example, paved sidewalks, ramps, and roads on which motorized wheel chairs can move). Low levels of development translate into malnutrition, an unsanitary environment, lack of prenatal care and trained attendance in childbirth, and the absence of rehabilitation services. The point of the distinction between disability and handicap is precisely the difference in conditions between a wealthy industrial country in the North and an impoverished developing country in the South. Nongovernmental organizations can provide services for the disabled but only governments can transform the built environment, for example by requiring architects to observe principles of universal design.[1]

Disability correlates directly with violence, armed conflict, and war. The incidence of disability soars during wartime when weapons, landmines, burns, poisoning, mutilation, and too often rape create a much higher incidence of injury. War zones also limit the availability of treatment for injuries, and delayed treatment may cause long-term disabilities. Wars create poverty by destroying markets, housing, transport, hospitals, and schools. It is instructive to contrast the experiences of amputees in Sierra Leone—with limited access to even the most primitive prosthetics—to that of disabled people in the North where disabled dancers, for example, are able to continue performing even in their wheelchairs.

The well-established association between disability and crime also relates to poverty. Research in the United States consistently finds that people with substantial disabilities suffer from violence, sexual abuse, and other crimes at rates four to ten times higher than that of the general population (Sorenson 1997). Crime rates are higher in poor (and poorly policed) neighborhoods, and crime impoverishes its victims.

In addition to broad social issues, personal hurdles confront all disabled women who find that safeguarding their privacy against both offhanded and deliberate violation requires continual vigilance and assertiveness. Insensitive physicians force disabled women to disrobe and display their different-looking bodies; they may perform medical exams with doors or curtains open and discuss information about their patients' sexual lives carelessly in public. People see these violations, deliberate or not, as coming from professional health authorities and as normalizing or legitimizing disrespectful attitudes toward the disabled.

Many disabled girls grow up with the message that the adult world of marriage and children is one that will always exclude them, that sex is for the healthy and whole, and that disabled women must give up the desire for love, physical closeness, and sexual relations (Marris 1996). Part of the negative response to sexuality in the disabled is the conservative concern with gene pools, a message used to effect by the eugenics movement (see chapter 6 on women's reproductive rights). Concern doubles when disabled people marry one another, although their disabilities may have no heritable characteristics. Disabled women who give birth may have a harder time proving their ability to mother and may face pressure to relinquish their children.

Society justifies its invasive custody over women with disabilities and the interference with their childbearing by stereotyping the disabled woman as a perpetually asexual child or elder. Control of disabled women's bodies, like the fertility control of women of color, is selective and not subtle. Men were not subject to the same sterilization laws that the eugenics movement introduced in the United States, which condemned so many women to childlessness. The law protected men on the grounds that men's bodily integrity must be respected.

Differences between North and South are also partly due to the presence or absence of political will to set priorities for the disabled and to adopt public health policies like the 1990 Americans with Disabilities Act. Currently, only 45 countries have adopted laws that deal with disability rights, according to UN officials (Rizvi 2006). Disability rights movements can and do influence policy. In addition to the charitable organizations created for disabled people, grassroots movements like Disabled in Action, Paralyzed Veterans of America, and Independent Living are nongovernmental organizations that disabled people control directly. The Independent Living movement established Independent Living centers in Brazil, Canada, Great Britain, and the United States (Malhotra 2001). People with disabilities have campaigned for workplaces built around disabled people's lives, doing away with discrimination in recruitment, pay, and promotion. They have also gained flexible working hours and individualized accommodations to ensure that work is accessible to people with different kinds of disability.

Flexibility/Agility/Performance

Disability marginalizes women whom society judges unable to conform to physical and mental norms. Emily Martin (1994) raises salient questions in her book about flexible bodies drawing attention to the use of the concept of flexibility in several unrelated fields including sports, corporate management, and immunology. The field of "extreme sports" sets new, higher standards for physical performance; and in the corporate world the buzzwords are agility and nimbleness. The implications for an analysis of the disabled are stunning.

The higher bars for flexibility and agility necessarily marginalize physically and mentally disabled people. Martin shows that flexibility, a concept that comes from systems theory and one that immunologists like to use when talking about parts of the immune system, is now widely applied in corporate culture to the workplace and to organizational structure. Flexibility contrasts with mechanical systems that are rigid, static, or in equilibrium. It means the ability to adjust continuously to change, to innovate, and incorporate failures. It also has a dark side that corporations talk less about: passivity, acquiescence, and the loss of security in the new "flexible" (temporary) workforce. Interestingly, many disabled people stress independence and their ability to adapt as sources of pride.

Immunologists see the human body as a good example of a flexible system, one that is loosely coupled (in contrast to tightly coupled mechanical systems). They characterize the human body as versatile because it is plastic and durable. The model for this portrait is a young, athletic male. The corporate world applies the concept of flexibility to both management and managers. For example, "the management of a global corporate culture that is adaptable and capable of dealing with rapid changes in the environment requires managers who are extremely flexible and can perform a wide range of functions" (Martin 1994, 145). It follows that training for total quality management, the common management term for this school of thought, consists of exercises like a leap into space from a 40-foot tower. CEOs call this empowered learning. Clearly, it is not for the disabled.

The concept of flexibility provides a link between individualism and conformity. Individualists reject the group behavior characteristic of trade unions, civil rights groups, and women's rights groups, which they call anachronistic and reactionary, deriding centralized union bureaucracies as rigid. By insisting on flexibility in decisionmaking, individualists are conforming to neoliberal ideology and justifying their selfish decisions on the libertarian grounds of free choice. Underneath this individualism is the same old corporate conformity and profit motive. Flexibility is a new term for an old practice—extracting more productivity from each worker at lower cost for the employer by making workers absorb more of the base expenses. In flextime, workers make their own hours; flexiplace means one works in an office or at home or in a hotel or at a cyberspace station in a café, library, or store. The good, flexible worker is nimble and agile like an acrobat on a high wire. She is also a temporary worker, available at a moment's notice and therefore insecure, without health insurance, with no paid leave, no bonuses, no opportunities for advancement, and no representation in the workplace (Martin 1994). Flexible jobs are temporary jobs, freeing employers of the obligation to pay pensions, or they are jobs filled by free-lance consultants on contract who must heat, light, and equip their own office, pay their own insurance in the absence of national programs (at individual rates higher than the group rates that employers can negotiate), and forgo pay for time off—whether for national holidays, personal vacations, or sick days.

The emphasis on bodily flexibility draws on sports, especially extreme sports. The new flexibility supplants the old demand for physical strength required of manual workers. Just when technology reduced the need for brawn and thus removed a physical barrier to the employment of women and disabled workers in some better paid jobs, a new barrier is erected, paradoxically one that demands physical agility for mental work. How can the disabled fit in the new flexible systems?

In terms of global corporate cultures, flexibility throws a negative light on traditional societies, which are stereotypically portrayed as rigid. Creating a new hierarchy of nations, flexibility casts the North as modern, civilized, urban (and its workers are flexible); the South is rigid, traditional, rural—and its workers? Well, in this vision only the very young and able-bodied who can adapt to constant change have a chance. Left behind are older or disabled workers—whatever their contributions to culture and society.

This trend to the demand for flexible bodies pushes public policy in the wrong direction—to an exclusive emphasis on employability—when we need a broader concern that places disability in the wider context of an economy's current and future labor needs. The focus should be on the workforce, not the worker, and on the general nature of work (Zola 1989).

The United Nations Division for Social Policy and Development has long discussed disability; the UN declared 1981 The International Year of Disabled Persons and 1983–1992 The United Nations Decade of Disabled Persons; and it maintains a Web site (http://esa.un.org/socdev/enable/search.htm) for persons with disabilities containing a database on international norms and standards. On 13 December 2006 the General Assembly adopted the Convention on the Rights of Persons with Disabilities (http://www.un.org/esa/socdev/enable/) to promote, protect, and ensure the full and equal enjoyment of all human rights and fundamental freedoms by all persons with disabilities, and to promote respect for their inherent dignity. Although it proclaims equality between men and women, the convention makes no special analysis of intersectionality, the overlap of sexism, racism, and other prejudices. Many groups concerned with human rights and disability—governmental and nongovernmental—participated in the process of drafting the UN convention, but women's health movements do not appear to have played a prominent role.[2]

The disability rights movement attempts to press for better access to employment for people with psychiatric disabilities. In the United States, the Kennedy family started a movement for the mentally retarded, motivated by the plight of a mentally retarded sister. But this is a field where the nature of the incapacity makes it almost impossible for people who suffer from mental disability to organize themselves for better treatment. As a result improvements have come, at a slow pace, from sympathetic crusaders.

Mental health

According to WHO (2001), mental health and mental illness are not opposites but substantially different states. Mental health implies that individual, group, and environmental factors work effectively together to ensure subjective well-being, optimal development and use of mental abilities, and achievement of goals consistent with justice and equality.

Table 7.1 Ten leading causes of disability worldwide, 1990

	Total (millions)	Percent of total
All Causes	472.7	
1 Unipolar major depression	50.8	10.7
2 Iron-deficiency anemia	22.0	4.7
3 Falls	22.0	4.6
4 Alcohol use	15.8	3.3
5 Chronic obstructive pulmonary disease	14.7	3.1
6 Bipolar disorder	14.1	3.0
7 Congenital anomalies	13.5	2.9
8 Osteoarthritis	13.3	2.8
9 Schizophrenia	12.1	2.6
10 Obsessive-compulsive disorders	10.2	2.2

Source: Murray, C.J.L. and A.D. Lopez. *The global burden of disease*. Cambridge, MA: Harvard University Press, 1996.

Mental disorders are recognized illnesses diagnosed medically, resulting in significant impairment of thinking processes, perceptions, moods and feelings, ways of interacting with others, and the environment. Although the positive definition of mental health is welcome, the contrast with mental illness as a substantially different state overemphasizes the difference of the mentally disabled and does not acknowledge the continuum of behavior in varied cultural contexts. It also takes as given the assignment of diagnoses overlooking the influence of racism, sexism, and class prejudice. Worldwide, the burden of disability is enormous, and the contribution of psychiatric diseases to the total global disease burden was 10.5 percent in 1990 (the most recent data available) and is estimated to rise to 15 percent by 2020 (www.hsph.harvard.edu/Organizations/bdu/GBDseries.html accessed 6 April 2007) (see table 7.1).

Framing Mental Illness

Of all the subjects covered in this book none shows as clearly as mental illness the egregious consequences for women of economic inequality, sexism, heterosexism, homophobia, racism, class prejudice, and the stigma of disability.

The field of psychiatry is ideologically riven, and the consequences of these disagreements play out in diagnosis and treatment of women's mental illnesses. The common theories of disease causation (see chapter 2) have parallels in the field of mental illness. Psychiatrists make use of the germ theory, which holds that specific disease agents cause specific illnesses, to explain such mental conditions as the psychosis of late stage syphilis. Genetic theory, which describes illnesses as inherited or genetically determined, can explain some forms of mental illness and mental retardation (for example, Huntington's chorea and Down's syndrome). Some psychiatrists use the theory of multifactorial causation, which holds that diseases have not one but several causes, to explain aberrant behavior associated with cardiovascular disease (Type A), as well as the environmental and social causes of the neuroses, and brain tumors that are the physical causes of some abnormal behavior. Lifestyle theory singles out deviant behaviors to explain addictions, domestic violence, and child abuse, especially over generations. Social production theory examines class, race, and gender subordination to explain some mental illnesses like depression associated with economic exploitation and political repression. This account is more or less the chronological development of etiology. Mental health practitioners too often base their treatment on the contribution of a single theory.

Three distinct models of care for the mentally ill follow from the etiological theories. The medical model (germ theory, genetics) relies on biomedical psychiatry using drugs, electroshock therapy, hospitalization, and surgery. The social model (multifactorial causation, lifestyle) encompasses medical approaches to situate mental illness in the community, but community-based care is an ideal rarely realized in practice. The public health model attempts to integrate prevention and care for the mentally ill into public health services, but the lack of trained personnel and scarce resources for psychiatric medication frequently thwart the attempts. Critics claim that the public health model rarely takes into account race, class, and sex biases. Still the public health approach is important in Third World countries with few resources available to construct separate facilities for the mentally ill. Although descriptive of current therapeutic approaches, models are not explanatory; they do not explain what causes psychiatric illness and disease or even why some people remain healthy while others fall ill under the same conditions.

Psychiatric epidemiology may show the distribution of illnesses in various groups, but mortality and morbidity rates by "race" are ambiguous. They could mean that there are biological differences, sociological differences, or environmental differences among the groups. Or the explanation could lie outside medicine altogether. The body of psychiatric literature in Africa contains very few studies of women. In the colonial era, this gap was attributable to the belief of European doctors in the protective function of traditional societies (the "happy native" theory); and, because more men than women migrated to towns, most women remained under the "protection" of families. Europeans also believed that African women reacted mildly to stressful situations that caused anguish to women in Europe: for example, they believed that African women do not experience grief at the death of a child. When colonial physicians did find signs of mental misery, usually among men who left home to find paid work, they mistook maladjustment to subhuman living and working conditions for an inability to deal with modern ways.

The failure of postcolonial medicine to investigate mental illness in women is more difficult to explain: other priorities, the small medical corps, an underdeveloped health care system, and the low status of women all contributed. Some NGOs try to supplement public services by offering help to women in distress. The International Rescue Committee worked in Tanzanian camps with refugees from Burundi counseling survivors of sexual and gender-based violence in drop-in centers (Nduna and Rude 1998). Hotline is a Thai center that offers counseling and psychotherapy over the telephone. Started in 1985 in Bangkok and then expanded to other parts of the country, Hotline added other services, such as personal visits, self-defense classes, and a magazine (Tantiwiramanond and Pandey 1991).

The field of addiction—to alcohol, tobacco, and drugs—demonstrates the lack of consensus in mental health theory and the consequences for women of the way illness is framed. Addiction ricochets between the poles of biomedical explanation (alcoholism is a disease) and lifestyle theories (alcoholism is self-destructive behavior, a moral failure). In 1989 the obstetrics department of the Medical University of South Carolina began testing the urine of pregnant women whom they suspected of using cocaine. They turned positive tests results over to the local prosecutor and police who arrested women, sometimes at the hospital just after giving birth (Greenhouse 2000). Medical organizations criticized the practice as criminalizing a public health problem better addressed by treatment than by punishing pregnant drug abusers. The U.S. Supreme Court considered the drug tests warrantless and amounted to unconstitutional searches in *Ferguson v. City of Charleston* (http://www.aclu.org/reproductiverights/lowincome/12511res20001101.html accessed 1 April 2007). According to South Carolina's law, a fetus is legally a child so a woman who is taking drugs, drinking alcohol, or engaging in other behaviors that pose a risk to the fetus can be prosecuted for child abuse. Police charged a woman in Georgia in 1999 with capital murder for the death, moments after birth, of one of a pair of premature twins; the mother tested positive for cocaine and methamphetamine and had received no prenatal care. By 2000 police departments had prosecuted some 200 women in 30 states on various legal theories of "fetal abuse." Although drug use crosses all racial and class lines, the police have overwhelmingly targeted and arrested poor women of color for using drugs while pregnant.

Another example of the lack of consensus in the analysis of mental illness is the treatment of sexuality that falls outside heterosexist norms. Many psychiatrists regard homosexuality as an illness requiring treatment (and until 1973 the DSM listed homosexuality as a psychiatric disorder). A study of the treatment of lesbians and gay men in the South African military in the apartheid era and found that homosexuals were barred from the permanent force and homosexual conscripts were referred to health professionals for medical treatment, sometimes including electric shock and conversion therapy (de Gruchy and Lewin 2001). Conversion therapy is an attempt to convert a person from a homosexual to a heterosexual orientation, although no evidence exists that such therapies can change sexual orientation, and the field of mental health does not support the use of conversion therapy.

Stressful Life Events: Poverty

Some of the psychiatric literature recognizes the importance of stressful life events such as death of a spouse, divorce, marital separation, jail term, death of a close family member, personal injury or illness, marriage, fired at work, marital reconciliation, retirement, and pregnancy. This recognition arises from research in industrial countries, not in Africa, Asia, or Latin America. In African countries where death in pregnancy is a more frequent occurrence than in Europe or North America, childbirth is associated with death and may be far more stressful than losing a job. In Benin, pregnant women say they have one foot in the grave, "birth is an experience between life and death. You don't know whether you will survive or not" (de Koninck 1998, 160). Missing altogether from the life events scale is burial: questionnaires should ask, were you able to bury your loved one with proper ceremonies? Burial is a major issue wherever civil wars provoke flight, making final rites impossible. The tragedy of September 11th 2001 finally brought home to Americans the importance of retrieving and identifying bodies, a rite that the public had recognized only in relation to prisoners of war and soldiers missing in battle.

Another issue missing from the inventory is poverty, which WHO's *World Mental Health* (Desjarlais, et al. 1995) links to a higher prevalence of psychiatric morbidity in women. Mental illness links to structural violence, which is the systemic violence that results in poverty, malnutrition, and social segregation. Poverty dampens the spirit and causes despair, causes families to lose their homes and become displaced, makes child death rates and mental retardation rates soar, leads to substance abuse, fans racial hatreds, contributes to abuse of women and children, leads to depression, severe mental illness, and suicide. Every study of mental illness since the Second World War (beginning with the work of Hollingshead and Redlich 1958) has shown a positive correlation between mental illness and social class: most illness is found in the lowest classes, making the association of mental illness and poverty clear. *World Mental Health* says more about poverty than mental illness as such, redressing the usual tendency to ignore poverty. The correlation of poverty and mental illness holds both North and South, as does the failure to provide adequate treatment.

When interviewers asked Ghanaian women about their health problems they spoke, not of reproductive health, but of psychosocial health problems, of worrying too much, which they linked to being tired, not sleeping, and having headaches (Avotri and Walters 1999). Women say they think too much, that they bear the entire responsibility for their children; and the financial insecurity they face adds to the uncertainties of their lives, leading them to work even longer hours. The behavior associated with worry sometimes became unusual—like talking to themselves loudly.

In the spring of 2002 the *New York Times* ran a series of articles on treatment of the mentally ill in New York City (Levy 2002a, 2002b, 2002c). For the 15,000 New Yorkers who cannot pay for private services—the poor, many black and Latino—treatment consists of residence in poorly maintained and understaffed adult homes. In the *Times* investigation these homes are institutions housing 60 to 430 "starkly ill people"; the homes lacked sufficient personnel, facilities, supplies, and equipment to protect residents from destructive and self-destructive behavior, or even to give the most basic routine care to prevent fatal outcomes from seizures and appendicitis. The *Times* documented 946 deaths from 1995 through 2001; 326 were of people under 60 years old. Fourteen residents committed suicide, one died of stab wounds inflicted by his roommate. State oversight is derisory; for example, the State Department of Health never enforced a 1994 law that requires homes to report all deaths. In these squalid, chaotic conditions, women are especially vulnerable to abuse and exploitation. At Seaport Manor, a home opened in Brooklyn, New York, in 1975 for 173 patients and housing 325 in 2002, prostitution and violence are common. Male and female residents trade sex for spending money, cigarettes, or drugs. Some residents sell crack openly to others, although drug abuse is a problem that leads to confinement. Pushers shake down fellow residents for their disability allowance.

The placement of the mentally ill in these facilities rather than in psychiatric hospitals dates back to the 1960s; a movement for deinstitutionalization pressed the states to close psychiatric hospitals, but local governments failed to provide the community services that the deinstitutionalization movement envisioned. New York State currently finances 25,000 beds in small group homes, supportive housing, and other residences, but these facilities are for the less ill, people who are able to manage their lives. The rest are divided between jails and profit-making adult homes that shelter patients that hospitals have discharged. For $28 a day per resident, the homes are supposed to provide meals, activities, and supervision and bring in psychiatric and medical care as needed. New York City takes the money from residents' monthly Social Security disability checks to pay the homes' operators (Levy 2002c). Several of the homes became "Medicaid mills": in order to bill Medicaid and Medicare, operators and health care providers pressured residents to undergo treatment, even surgery, they neither needed nor understood. The warehousing of the mentally ill in jails, where they receive little or no psychiatric care and where guards and other inmates subject them to abuse, has also finally surfaced following several suicides (see, for example, the website of Prison Reform Trust, a U.K. charity, www.prisonreformtrust.org.uk/subsection.asp?id=315 accessed 10 January 2007).

A little discussed class aspect of deinstitutionalization is that the shift from publicly funded state institutions to small, privately managed group homes has also entailed a transfer of public service workers—many of them women—from relatively well paid positions that carried benefits to community service jobs that are poorly paid with no benefits. Public employee unions all over the United States fought against deinstitutionalization for this reason, and in many states they succeeded in stopping or slowing down any movement to close or downsize facilities (Kafka 2003).

In exploring reasons for the deplorable situation in the adult homes, the *Times* pointed out that the mentally ill "are among the most powerless of all populations, lacking the political influence to demand change and, in the case of adult home residents, having few advocates to take up their cause" unlike the homeless (Levy 2002d). The only group that regularly tries to assist residents is the nonprofit Coalition of Institutionalized Aged and Disabled. In July 2001 the Coalition filed a complaint with the Health Department seeking an investigation of excessive and unnecessary eye surgery performed on residents.

Mental Disability Rights International (MDRI, http://www.mdri.org/), a nonprofit based in Washington, DC, found children with disabilities hidden and wasting away, near death, in Romania's adult psychiatric facilities—teenagers weighing no more than 27 pounds, some tied down with bed sheets, their arms and legs twisted and left to atrophy. In a two-year investigation in Turkey MDRI detailed human rights abuses perpetrated against children and adults with psychiatric and developmental disabilities in psychiatric facilities, orphanages, and rehabilitation centers where the use of electroconvulsive treatment on psychiatric patients as young as nine-years-old without the use of anesthesia is widespread. The investigators also found evidence of children dying from starvation, dehydration, and lack of medical care in residential rehabilitation centers. In Paraguay, MDRI and the Center for Justice and International Law settled with the Paraguayan government to end the improper detention of hundreds of people in the country's state-run psychiatric hospital. Filed with the Inter-American Commission on Human Rights of the Organization of American States, the settlement is the first agreement in Latin America to guarantee the rights of patients to live and receive mental health services in the community.

The focus on biomedical psychiatric diagnoses coupled with the neglect of factors like gender, race, and class has led to the arbitrary attribution of the radically different diagnoses of insanity, criminality, and political protest. Four examples will suffice to demonstrate the confusion of diagnoses and the role of poverty (all of the people discussed here are white).

Andrew Goldstein, who had a ten-year history of schizophrenia and psychiatric hospitalizations, shoved Kendra Webdale in front of a Manhattan subway train in 1999, killing her (Winerip 1999). Too poor to afford a lawyer, the court appointed one; the jury rejected his insanity plea and convicted him of murder as a criminal. Eight years later, after intensive psychiatric treatment while incarcerated, Goldstein pleaded guilty to murder (Hartocollis 11 October 2006). Andrea Yates drowned her five children in their bath in 2001; she had made two suicide attempts in 1999 and was hospitalized several times for schizophrenia. Texas law does not equate mental illness with insanity nor can a defendant enter a plea of guilty and insane. The standard for the insanity plea is no knowledge of wrongdoing. As Yates said she was a "bad mother," indicating that she knew that punishment awaited her when she called the police, a jury found her guilty of capital murder (Bard 2002); a court overturned the verdict on appeal. A jury acquitted John Hinckley who tried to kill President Reagan in 1981, finding him not guilty by reason of insanity; Hinckley's parents were wealthy and able to hire an expensive lawyer to defend him (Vatz 2006). In contrast, Lynette "Squeaky" Fromme, a poor woman who tried to assassinate President Ford, was convicted as a criminal, although she was a follower of Charles Manson's crazed white supremacist cult. Political protest is not a category of criminality in the United States—protestors are convicted as either criminals or insane, and a successful insanity plea depends on the ability to pay a first-class lawyer.

Mental Health in War Zones

The direct effects of conflict, which lead to collective trauma, are the destruction of homes, schools, and workplaces. The cumulative effects that reinforce and prolong trauma are wide-scale loss of human capital, death, and disability. Emergent effects include scapegoating, rejection of rape victims and "war babies," and ongoing violence against women. Important to recovery from trauma are the interactions of direct, cumulative, and emergent effects that exacerbate suffering. In addition certain transgenerational effects, which carry the trauma to later generations, leave deep scars: the weaving of cultural narratives of war and the creation of identities of victimization, as well as the rejection of raped women and their children.

Feminists criticize the models of treatment for victims of trauma that psychiatrists originally developed to treat (mostly male) combatants after the Vietnam War (Giller 1998; Sideris 2003). This treatment, which included medication, early intervention, desensitization, and cognitive behavioral techniques, is based on the symptoms of post-traumatic stress disorder (PTSD). Psychiatrists revised the definition of PTSD in 1994 as follows: "The person experienced, witnessed, or was confronted with an event or events that involved actual or threatened death or serious injury or a threat to the physical integrity of self or others and which evoked intense fear, helplessness or horror." (DSM IV 1994) This definition broadens traumatic exposure well beyond the original concept that described the reaction of individuals to discrete violent incidents related to one's self and one's comrades.

PTSD accounts for short-term, acute trauma (like motor vehicle accidents and single incidents of assault), but it does not account well for prolonged repeated trauma (like sustained child sex abuse, concentration camp life, ongoing domestic violence, or repeated torture). And although PTSD accounts for individual trauma like accidents, assaults, and single acts of rape, it does not account well for collective trauma such as ethnic cleansing, death squads, and terrorism.

In considering the impact of civil war on women, the collective aspects of trauma are of greatest concern. Civilians (mostly women, children, and the elderly) are embedded in a social and cultural order, and the trauma they experience is related to the disruption of basic relations of production and reproduction. The immediate effects are population displacement that breaks up families and destroys villages; personal and economic insecurity; and human rights abuses. Long-term effects include the unraveling of social roles and rituals of social structure, the silencing of victims and witnesses, and the loss of trust in neighbors and others.

Important gender issues derive from the definition of women's well-being (more so than men's) as linked to having a social place. Social dislocation has an impact on women's access to material resources, on their social status, and their power. Women's issues for the treatment of trauma revolve around sexuality—fertility and infertility, contraceptive use, protection against sexually transmitted diseases—and certain beliefs such as that rape is "spirit injury," women are property, raped women are "damaged goods," female sexuality is a commodity, and rape dishonors the family.

Gendered treatment is not yet a part of the medical model. Medics can identify male combatants in need of care in the command structure and refer them to veterans' facilities. Most women and children in war-torn countries find it more difficult to seek and receive treatment (especially for rape). More useful is the social model of treatment that focuses on social reconstruction, the reestablishment of economic networks, and reparations.

Diversity and Difference

Disability and mental illness are but two instances of diversity and difference. Women, like men, come in all shapes, sizes, and colors; we are of diverse ethnicities and a range of sexual preferences. Yet judgment against a stereotypical norm is more severe for women than men. These norms and stereotypes are inimical to the appreciation of difference and the elimination of diversities that reflect inequality; they negatively affect women's well-being and health. The roots of the norms to which women adapt are found in political philosophy, in the origins of conformity, and in policies of exclusion. The heritage of Western political philosophy reveals the consistent rejection of diversity, despite the multicultural nature of modern societies. Multinational corporations use conformity to promote their products and thereby perpetuate rigid norms.

Origins of Conformity

Notions of identity, especially national identity, are changing under the pressures of immigration, the dissolution of some nation-state boundaries in large communities such as the European Union, and the fragmentation of other nation-states into smaller entities of ethnic homogeneity. Too many commentators frame the discussion of difference in cultural terms that disregard the political foundations of conformity.

Two European women pushed for women's equal rights—Olympe de Gouges (1735–1793), author of the Declaration of the Rights of Woman and the Female Citizen, and Mary Wollstonecraft (1759–1797) who wrote *A Vindication of the Rights of Woman*. Both were responding to contemporary French ideas of education and equality, de Gouges to the revolutionary Declaration of the Rights of Man and of the Citizen and Wollstonecraft to *Émile* by Jean Jacques Rousseau (1712–1778), which discusses education for boys. Wollstonecraft argued that what appeared to be the nature of woman was actually a consequence of the miseducation of women—a miseducation that men imposed on them. The lack of equal education for women condemns them to dependence on men and conformity to male stereotypes of women as ignorant and irrational.

Neither de Gouges nor Wollstonecraft proved able to persuade followers of Thomas Hobbes (1588–1679) of the need to constrain individual competition in order to construct a cooperative and egalitarian society. Hobbes' view of individualism prevailed in the popular mind, reinforced in the nineteenth century by a vulgar interpretation of Charles Darwin (1809–1882) that reduced evolutionary theory to a cliché—the survival of the fittest. One curious aspect of Hobbesian competition as the philosophical basis for capitalist economies is its transformation into a positive ideology of individualism. Individualism, which should not be confused with individuality, is the doctrine that governmental or social regulation should not restrict individual freedom in economic enterprise. Ironically Hobbes' theory leads to conformism and to conventional behavior for without normative arrangements, a society organized in the way Hobbes describes would descend into anarchy.

Individualism equates nonconformism with personal maladjustment. Individuals who fail to fit into established roles and norms—roles and norms that the powerful in society establish—are a threat to the well-being of society. Examples from women's history, which is a history of subordination and resistance, illustrate this point. Over time society has redefined women's nonconformism variously as giving birth to illegitimate children (and unwed mothers were imprisoned or institutionalized); as divorce, which certain religions and state laws do not allow; as lesbianism (homosexuality and sodomy are still against the law in many places and condemned in religious doctrines); and as mental illness (nonconforming women were institutionalized as mentally ill). In the process of equating unbridled competition with masculine attributes of rugged individualism, society embraced inequality as the natural order of the universe.

The commitment to appreciating diversity in the United States emerged out of the struggle against racism, and the word diversity became important when the Supreme Court ruled in 1978 in *Bakke v. Board of Regents* that considerations of race in university admissions were acceptable if they served the interests of diversity. Note that the Court did not assert that universities could give preference in admissions because society had previously discriminated against black people. The Court said that universities had a legitimate interest in racial diversity in the way they had a legitimate interest in geographic diversity. This decision connected two unrelated concepts—diversity and race—and associated the commitment to diversity with the struggle against racism (Michaels 2006).

> Our commitment to diversity has thus redefined the opposition to discrimination as the appreciation (rather than the elimination) of difference. So with respect to race, the idea is not just that racism is a bad thing (which of course it is) but that race itself is a good thing. And what makes it a good thing is that it's not class. We love race—we love identity—because we don't love class . . . A world where some of us don't have enough money is a world where the differences between us present a problem: the need to get rid of inequality or to justify it. A world where some of us are black and some of us are white—or bi-racial or Native American or transgendered—is a world where the differences between us present a solution: appreciating our diversity. (Michaels 2006, 20)

Class, racial, and gender inequalities of power and resources shape social problems and generate conflicts between the powerful and powerless. Employers rely on the dynamics of sexism, racism, and class prejudice to get cheap labor, and the exploitation and discrimination that workers experience lead to alienating behavior, social alienation, even criminality and deviance.

The Uses and Abuses of Difference

The importance of these worldviews to women becomes clear in a discussion of the impact of beauty myths on women's health and independence. One of the biggest myths is that women must want to embody beauty and men must want to possess women who embody it. This embodiment is an imperative for women and an option for men, a gender difference that sociobiologists say is both necessary and natural because it is biological, sexual, and evolutionary. Feminists criticize this essentialist position, yet many women believe that a woman's access to power lies in her physical appearance; and underlying this belief is the Hobbesian vision of a society in competition for power, privilege, and prestige. Naomi Wolf (1990) claims that men determine beauty politically and economically. She argues that as women in industrial societies emerged successfully in many new arenas (higher education, the trades, and the professions), the focus on and demand for beauty became more intense, attacking women's private sense of self and creating new barriers to accomplishment. By making beauty a premise of women's identity, society ensures women's vulnerability to outside approval, one more cord that binds women to social conventions and conformity. Wolf sees this increasing obsession with beauty as a backlash to the women's liberation movement.

Culture of course plays a role in our perceptions of normality, beauty, and ugliness. Cultural preoccupation with how we look assaults the appreciation and expression of women's diversity. Social concerns with appearance affect our physical and emotional health; depression and low self-esteem follow from attempts to conform to impossibly idealized standards of beauty. More important, from the perspective of women's health movements, these superficial concerns distract us from activities to improve social conditions. The power of appearance pushes people to assimilate, it assaults diversity in beauty, and it affects our self-worth. It also persuades women to purchase products and procedures that manufacturers assure them will improve their chances of success. Technological advancements in breast enhancement and cosmetic surgery, which carry serious health risks, change our perceptions of how we can achieve beauty. They assault our expression of diversity even as they destroy health and well-being. As these norms migrate across the globe, the United States is exporting American beauty ideals to other countries. Skin-whitening products, for example, are popular in Asia and Africa, despite the dangerous consequences of mercury-based creams, which are linked to leukemia (Fuller 2006).

When one learns of the vast commercial interests vested in marketing beauty, profit seems more likely than culture to drive the (changing) norms of beauty. Cosmetic surgery alone is a $15 billion industry in the United States (Kuczynski 2006). Industries like clothing, cosmetics, diet, and fitness set the beauty standard, changing fashions every season and employing sophisticated advertising techniques to convince women that they need to purchase these goods. The second wave of the women's movement in the United States initially focused on issues of a single standard of beauty and pressures for conformity: women protested against the Miss America contest where they burned brassieres, a symbol of the breast-obsessed nation. They spurned makeup, made being fat a feminist issue, and protested against Playboy—both the magazine and the club and more generally against the humiliation of women waiting on tables while wearing revealing clothing.

A single standard of beauty suppresses diversity (Zones 1997). Society uses the beauty standard to enforce conformity, push assimilation, and reward conventionality. The single standard of beauty and the pressures to conform to it are pervasive in health care. Nonconforming women are objects of discrimination and prejudicial treatment by health care providers. Health workers who behave in these biased ways are conformists, consciously or unconsciously upholding the values of conventional behavior, as when they mistreat lesbians (Stevens 1998) or press women cancer patients to undergo reconstructive breast surgery. Most of the content of health education consists of admonishments to conform to normative behavior.

Obesity and Wasting

The tyranny of conformism and a single standard of beauty are especially harmful to women when we consider the question of ideal weight. In the North we spend $50 billion a year to lose weight and to make ourselves look thinner or more like the established norm. The tyranny of conformism also leads some young women into anorexia and bulimia.

.The beauty standard for ideal weight is not fixed: it changes over time (the better to sell new products and services, no doubt). Twenty years ago models weighed 8 percent less than the average American woman; today they weigh 23 percent less and are much thinner than the average American woman who weighs 144 pounds and wears between a size 12 and 14. After six high-profile deaths of Brazilian models from anorexia in 2006, the fashion industries of Spain and France decided to ban underweight models (defined as having a body mass index of less than 18) from their runways (Wilson 2007). The American industry resisted. A recent psychological study found that girls who spend time looking at models in fashion magazines are more likely to experience an eating disorder in the next five years. The clothing industry propagates the image of the thin model beyond fashion magazines to toys and entertainment: grotesquely disproportioned Barbie dolls are credited with introducing a new body image to Brazilian girls and women (Rohter 2007).

Women in North America and Europe seem to be subject, in varying degrees, to perpetual dieting, compulsive exercising, or the pressure to do both. Nutrition education programs try to change individual behavior, but obesity, like hunger, appears to be more than an individual issue. Most people cannot affect societal aspects of obesity such as the lack of healthy food choices at work or in the community. Many poor people have few choices: a healthy lifestyle in an impoverished neighborhood is not a matter of self-determination.

Worldwide women are converging toward one standard of beauty—thin, tall, and white (Zones 1997). Although everyone in the North is exposed to similar societal pressures to be thin, only a small percentage develops eating disorders. One explanation is that girls and women who succumb to eating disorders are usually prompted by extreme career pressures, or have some underlying emotional or physical vulnerability (Brody 2000). Another view is that anorexia disrupts mental functions and acts on the brain not unlike an addiction (Brown 2006). Ironies abound: the rate of obesity is rising in the United States and Europe, even as some people in these societies are striving to be as thin as possible. Meanwhile the impoverished queue for food at charitable distribution centers and soup kitchens are unable to meet the needs of the hungry at their doors. Bellows (2003) calls these deprivations "food violences" and laments their structured invisibility.

Identity, defined in terms of appearance (skin color, masculinity and femininity, and clothing that marks ethnic or religious affiliation), is the least important thing about us and the most talked about. Our real problem is economic difference that we have started to regard as similar to cultural difference.

So now we are urged to be more respectful of poor people and to stop thinking of them as victims, since to treat them as victims is condescending—it denies them their "agency." And if we can stop thinking of the poor as people who have too little money and start thinking of them instead as people who have too little respect, then it is our attitude toward the poor, not their poverty, that becomes the problem to be solved (Michaels 2006, 22).

If we think of inequality as a consequence of our prejudices rather than as a consequence of our social system, we turn the project of creating a more egalitarian society into the project of getting people to stop being racist, sexist, and classist homophobes.

Social Inclusion and Universalism

The final section of this book tries to make sense of the philosophical and political underpinnings of conformity and the exclusion of those who are different from the dominant majority. Social inclusion is the goal of the new universalism proposed here. To understand the concept of social inclusion, it is necessary to trace briefly its origins in French discussions of the excluded.[3] The *exclus* were people excluded from employment-based social security systems—the disabled, suicidal, aged, abused children, and substance abusers. In the 1980s the *exclus* were more generally the socially disadvantaged, products of new social problems such as unemployment, ghettoization, and changed family life. Provisions of the old welfare state were not successful in inserting these individuals and groups into mainstream society (de Haan 1998).

In France, the paradigm of social inclusion is one of solidarity, after Jean-Jacques Rousseau (1712–1778),[4] and exclusion is the rupture of a social bond between the individual and society that is cultural and moral (de Haan 1998). In the United States social inclusion is a paradigm of individual responsibility, after Thomas Hobbes (1588–1679);[5] social exclusion reflects discrimination, the drawing of group distinctions that deny individuals full access to or participation in society. American commentators often find the causes of exclusion in unenforced rights and market failures. In Great Britain, the paradigm is that of hierarchical power, after Max Weber (1864–1920);[6] social exclusion is a consequence of the formation of group monopolies that restrict the access of outsiders through social closure. The British literature describes four dimensions of social exclusion: exclusion from adequate income or resources, labor market exclusion, service exclusion, and exclusion from social relations (Richmond 2002).

The increasing number of studies of social exclusion in the literature requires an explanatory context, which Jock Young, the British criminologist, provides. Young (1999) sees the transition from modernity to late modernity as a movement from an inclusive to an exclusive society, that is, from a society that accented assimilation and incorporation to one that separates and excludes. This erosion of the inclusive world of the modernist period involved processes of disaggregation in the sphere of community (the rise of individualism) and in the sphere of work (the transformation of the labor market). Both processes are the result of market forces and their transformation by the human actors involved (Dixon 2001).

In the context of the industrialized world, the transformation of late modernity occurs first in labor markets that are fragmented, creating a society in which only a central but shrinking core of citizens enjoys secure, well-paid employment. A secondary labor market provides temporary work that is often poorly paid. A section of the population, namely the excluded, is superfluous to the functioning of late capitalism and routinely denied the privileges of even this precarious existence (Dixon 2001). This exclusion is structural and may take one of two forms in the global South: instability, where civil order is maintained but relations between dominant groups are unstable, and warlordism, where hegemonic vacancy is manifested in violent civil disorder (Gore 1994).

In some countries citizenship is a prerequisite, not only for political inclusion in society, but also for access to jobs and benefits. Whereas some liberal democracies have moved steadily from citizenship to personhood when allocating social rights, the volatile world economy and the events of September 11th 2001 have resulted in anti-immigrant sentiment and new legislation to curb access to social investments such as job training and access to the labor market (Fix and Laglagaron 2002). The citizenship debates are pertinent to the global South because of research on the way entitlements are attached to affiliation or social identity (viz. Ekeh 1975; Gore 1994; Mamdani 1996).

On what terms are the *exclus* to be integrated? All three paradigms (solidarity, individual responsibility, and hierarchical power) lend themselves to the neoliberal model of privatization, although the French paradigm implies the nation's responsibility—not just the government's responsibility but also that of all members of society. All three paradigms lead to dependence on private, charitable provision of services.

World Bank publications articulate the neoliberal paradigm most clearly. Social equity, in the Bank's vocabulary, is secondary and subordinate to the promotion of the private sector. The State's first task is to create the appropriate institutional foundations necessary for the proper functioning of market forces. The redistributional role of the State is conditional on its ability to fulfill its basic economic functions, which are to establish the foundations of lawfulness, maintain economic stability, and invest in social services and infrastructure (the rudiments of public health, universal primary education, and a minimal social safety net). The claim that "markets can provide a variety of private goods and services that in many countries have somehow wandered into the domain of public provision, such as higher education, curative health services, and pensions and other forms of insurance" tempers even that minimal provision (World Bank 1997, 59–60). The Bank's advice to countries with weak public institutions is to "assign high priority to finding ways to use markets and involve private firms and other nongovernmental providers in service delivery" (World Bank 1997, 60). It seems to me that the World Bank is using notions of equity and poverty reduction to legitimize the neoliberal agenda, that it is defining equity and poverty reduction in such a way as to promote and advance the neoliberal economic agenda. The World Bank has not begun to incorporate economic and social rights as understood in the United Nations Universal Declaration of Human Rights (Campbell 2000).

If policymakers were articulating concepts of social exclusion in order to ensure programs of social inclusion, there would be little debate. But it appears that neoliberals interpret social exclusion to reinforce political exclusion. The substitution of charities for State services subverts the democratic process by bypassing planning mechanisms and disempowering people in regimes that use an electoral process to determine national priorities (even if that process is only nominal). When the private sector sets the agenda, it is neither national nor nationwide but local and fragmented; the process undermines the authority of the State and substitutes the profit motive for intrinsic social values.

The struggle for redistribution is a political struggle because privatization, in the guise of public/private partnerships and State funding of charities, really takes power out of the hands of the people and gives it to unelected boards of corporations and philanthropies that are not accountable to anyone and certainly not answerable to an electorate. More than resources are being redistributed when privatization occurs, power is also being concentrated at the top. Charities that create programs for the *exclus* do not bring them into the democratic arena where they can participate in debates over national priorities and vote their preferences, but into an autocratic arena where philanthropists decide on which programs they wish to fund (what is good for them; "them" being deliberately ambiguous, referring either to philanthropists or to the target population). Yet political inclusion is central to—even a prerequisite for—social inclusion (Beall, Crankshaw, and Parnell 2002).

U.S. policymakers are not articulating concepts of social exclusion in order to reorient policy to reintegrate the excluded; evidence for this assertion comes from current budgets. The extensive defunding of State services and the funding of "faith-based" programs in the private sector are consistent with U.S. insistence on the withdrawal of the State from service provision. In the current philosophy in Washington, the Bush administration clearly desires social inclusion only for the macroeconomic stability it promises. In this instrumentalist perspective, equality is important to economic efficiency and effectiveness that Washington believes is greatest in the private sector. Greater equity is not a reflection of intrinsic values at the center of strategies.

In the global South, exclusion applies to practices and processes by which social collectivities monopolize (usually economic) opportunities. Powerful elites monopolize resources through the exclusion of foreign owners in key economic sectors and by periodically expelling international migrant workers (Gore 1994). Bureaucratic or business elites monopolize opportunities through the manipulation of identity. In this analysis, the elites are the beneficiaries of indigenization.

The *exclus* are either the whole of the global South, refugees, or people designated as aliens; and at another level, the *exclus* are women, female-headed households, pastoralists and hunter-gatherers, internally displaced persons, the rural poor, and minorities at risk of disease and death (Gore 1994). This analysis of just who is disadvantaged or marginalized is obviously problematic: if we add up these groups, beginning with women, who comprise at least 50 per cent of society, then we arrive at a large majority, which subverts the meaning of social exclusion (social exclusion makes sense only when speaking of no more than 15 per cent of the population). The absence of class analysis, which is at the heart of discussions of social exclusion, diverts attention from the idea that class encompasses more than income, that it involves economic, political, and social relationships, as well as concepts of ownership and property. The processes of dividing the South into those included in societies and those excluded are poorly understood, although some recent work is making progress in analyzing aspects of the marginalization and dispossession of communities in colonial and postcolonial societies (Jeeves and Kalinga 2002).

Poverty is more and more closely linked to exclusion (Gore 1994); poverty and social identity are interrelated, and both are relatively important determinants of exclusion. International development programs address problems of poverty rather than social exclusion. The poverty alleviation strategies of the international agencies have evolved over time, beginning in the 1950s with growth through industrialization, moving in the 1960s to agricultural intensification and trickle-down economic theories, to redistribution and a focus on meeting basic human needs in the 1970s. The 1980s saw the neoliberal push for structural adjustment, rollbacks of State services, and the use of charities to alleviate the poverty these policies aggravate. The 1990s brought a new consensus in favor of broad-based labor-intensive economic growth, human capital development, and social safety nets for the vulnerable (de Haan 1998). Many critics see more continuity than change in the strategies of the last two decades.

Is social inclusion the equivalent of poverty reduction? What does the concept of social exclusion add to the debates about poverty? Current definitions of poverty in the UN system range from UNDP's work on human development[7] to the World Bank's ranking of GNP per capita, an admittedly narrow measure. Amartya Sen's (1999) work on capabilities and entitlements has influenced the UNDP in particular. Sen sees the determinants of deprivation not in what people possess but in what hinders them from meeting social conventions, participating in social activities, and retaining self-respect.

Feminists have joined the debate to point out the feminization of poverty and to redefine concepts of national security to include aspects of human security (Heyzer 2001; UNDP 1994).[8] I mention this because the literature on social inclusion, especially about the global South, is so often blind to gender differences, as if men and women experience poverty or exclusion in the same ways. This omission is singular considering the focus on institutions and actors. The feminist literature on the impact of structural adjustment programs on women is clear about women bearing the brunt of these policies (Sparr 1994).

The term used in development circles that most closely corresponds to social exclusion is vulnerability, meaning insecurity, defenselessness, and exposure to risks and shocks (Chambers 1989; de Haan 1998). To my mind, the emphasis on vulnerability shifts the focus from structural exclusion to subjective perception, a change that depoliticizes the discussion. Social exclusion, with its focus on the societal mechanisms, institutions, and actors that cause deprivation, is a step forward from neoliberal preoccupations with individual attributes of the deprived.

In the North, the socially excluded represent 10 to 15 per cent of the population, but in the South, upward of 50 per cent of the population of many countries live in absolute poverty (46 per cent in sub-Saharan Africa are without access to safe water, 52 per cent are without access to sanitation, 35 percent are not expected to survive to age 40, 41 per cent of adults are illiterate, and 31 per cent of children under the age of five are underweight [UNDP 2000]). Where such a large majority is unable to meet basic needs or enjoy social rights, the social exclusion classification seems meaningless.

The concept of social exclusion may offer something new to those who work on developing countries, particularly in its focus on the institutional processes that lead to deprivation (De Haan and Maxwell 1998). Institutional processes are at the heart of the poverty debate, and the social exclusion framework helps to focus on the institutions and actors involved in the processes that cause deprivation and so has immediate implications for policy (Rodgers 1997). It seems to me that the applicability of social exclusion to the South is questionable for reasons additional to those already stated, namely North/South gaps, the likelihood of greater political exclusion in the South, and the continuing decreased provision of State services, leading to political instability as state authority is further undermined.

In the North where the *exclus* are a numerical minority, the majority contributes both materially and morally to social institutions into which the *exclus* can potentially be integrated. In the South, not only do the majority live in absolute poverty and deprivation, but social institutions are few and economies into which the poor can potentially be integrated are rarely viable. Social exclusion remedies are directed at the formal labor market, a solution that has little purchase in countries with large informal and subsistence sectors (de Haan and Maxwell 1998).

The equation of social exclusion with poverty is a problematic trend that focuses attention on the demand for services, away from the problems of supply. The equation also carries the implication that services are there for those who can afford to buy them, but in many countries such services do not exist, especially not outside the major cities. The equation further implies that poverty is an absolute barrier to a better quality of life that includes health and education services, but this is also untrue. Equitable social organization that includes the even distribution of assets and resources can ensure access to basic services even in the face of national, household, and individual poverty. Equitable distribution was the policy at various times for Algeria, Mozambique, Tanzania, and Zimbabwe, just as it was in postwar Britain before Margaret Thatcher took office. The effects of this approach to equality and universality of service delivery and coverage are demonstrated in data from an unpublished World Bank study presented by Khama Rogo.[9] Countries investing in and equitably redistributing primary health care had better health outcomes than countries that made no such investment, even twenty years after policies had changed and the original system had deteriorated. Simon Szreter, commenting after Rogo's presentation, estimated that the effect of such investment lasts for two generations, an estimate he based on studies of the National Health Service in the United Kingdom.

The paradigms of social exclusion do move analyses away from a single dimension—income and poverty—to an array of factors. In most of the literature pertaining to the North, multidimensional conceptualization emphasizes process and diminished capacities for work. The problem in the transfer of the paradigm to the South is that these dimensions are far too few and too narrow to account for extremely complex situations that encompass civil strife, drought, famine, and environmental degradation.

A Final Word

This discussion has moved from differences due to disability and mental illness to the political philosophies underlying the rejection of deviations from ever-changing but always narrow physical and behavioral norms. My purpose has been to distinguish concepts of cultural difference from structural divisions that create economic classes. A fixation on an internationalized standard of beauty has done much harm to women and led to preoccupation with other markers of identity. Women's health movements have wrestled with these issues, which have fragmented and splintered groups in every country, deflecting attention from basic class divisions. As economic inequalities widen, women have found it increasingly difficult to focus on the fundamental inequities of economic class. Women recognize that the sources or causes of gender discrimination in the South have deep roots in the legacies of colonial land law and the unresolved tensions between statutory and customary law (customary law often discriminates against women; statutory law discriminates against noncitizens). We have also identified the ways current economic, social, and political dislocations exacerbate gender discrimination. We now need to push analysis of intersectionality much farther and dissect the ways those in power manipulate identities to distort our agenda, distracting women's health movements from efforts to eliminate class distinctions that are at the bottom of gender inequity and account for so much of women's ill health.

NOTES

Chapter One   Women Organizing: Activism Worldwide

1. In nongovernmental organizations (NGO status is a prerequisite), women organized forums around the four world women's conferences (1975 in Mexico, 1980 in Copenhagen, 1985 in Nairobi, 1995 in Beijing), the 1992 Earth Summit in Rio de Janeiro, the 1993 Human Rights Conference in Vienna, the 1994 Conference on Population and Development in Cairo, and the 1995 Social Summit in Copenhagen.
2. The Vatican published a collection of words and phrases that it says are code for anti-Catholic sentiments with terms like "gender" and "reproductive rights," supposedly used for pro-abortion propaganda. The Vatican publication, which includes 74 terms about family and life (WGNRR 2003b 42), is part of a new attack on women's reproductive rights, especially the agenda negotiated at the Cairo Conference.
3. The choice to focus on local and national level movements reflects my (ultimately frustrating) 12-year experience as a UN staff member with UNICEF and WHO. For a review of women's movements at the international level see Harcourt 2006 and Antrobus 2004.
4. See Eschle and Stammers (2000) for the distinctions among transnational advocacy networks, network organizations, and social movements.
5. Not all women's movements are feminist, meaning the critique of male bias and the examination of women's subordination. Feminism, a term first used in Europe at the end of the nineteenth century and publicized by Simone de Beauvoir in *The Second Sex*, has many interpretations (socialist, radical, lesbian, cultural, women of color). This book does not insist on such distinctions among women's movements.
6. Women belonging to 10 political parties formed the National Women's Coalition in 1996. The Coalition promotes women's equitable participation in the political life of Nicaragua and developed a "Minimum Agenda" as a means of promoting women's participation in the electoral process (United Nations Press Release 2001).
7. The Hindu Marriage Act (1955), the Hindu Succession Act and the Hindu Adoption and Maintenance Act (1956), followed by the Dowry Prohibition Act (1961), were collectively known at the Hindu Code Bills; originally designed to give equal property rights to women, abolish customary law, and specify grounds for divorce, the Constituent Assembly passed a watered down version, more symbolic than substantive (Som 1994).
8. The woman question, concerning private property, control of material assets, and woman's relation to man within families and society, was a major subject of debate within the social democratic and communist organizations of the late-nineteenth and early-twentieth centuries.

9. In 1922 Egyptians assumed responsibility for their internal affairs, but the British retained authority in foreign affairs and kept a military presence in Egypt (Badran 1995).

10. APRA is a left-wing social democratic political party that won 22.6 percent of the popular vote and 36 out of 120 seats in the Congress of the Republic at the legislative elections held on 9 April 2006, and the party's presidential candidate, Alan García, won 22.6 percent of the vote and went on to win the second round on 4 June 2006 with 52.6 percent. It remains to be seen whether he will continue to implement the program he inaugurated in his first presidency in 1985.

11. Philadelphians established the Society for the Relief of Free Negroes Unlawfully Held in Bondage in 1775, and the British organized the Committee for the Abolition of the Slave Trade in 1787.

12. See the literature on women's ways of knowing; for example Goldberger et al. 1996.

13. In Spanish, *Red de Salud de las Mujeres Latinoamericanas y del Caribe* (RSMLAC).

14. The first convened in 1977 in Rome, the second in 1980 in Hanover, the third in 1981 in Geneva, the fourth in 1984 in Amsterdam, the fifth in 1987 in Costa Rica, the sixth in 1990 in Manila, the seventh in 1993 in Kampala, the eighth in 1996 in Rio de Janeiro, the ninth in 2002 in Toronto, and the tenth in 2005 in New Delhi.

Chapter Two   The Global Context

1. Adopted at the Fourth World Conference on Women, held in Beijing, China, 4–15 September 1995 (UN 1996).

2. The World Trade Organization is not part of the UN system; it grew out of the Uruguay Round of trade talks. WTO is a place where member governments sort out the trade problems they face with each other. At its heart are the WTO agreements, negotiated and signed by the bulk of the world's trading nations. But the WTO is not just about liberalizing trade (http://www.wto.org/english/thewto_e/whatis_e/tif_e/fact1_e.htm accessed 12 June 2006).

3. The G8 nations are the major industrial powers: Canada, France, Germany, Italy, Japan, Russia, Great Britain, and the United States. Russia is a relatively recent addition to the G-7.

4. The U.S. Congress first passed restrictions on financing abortions abroad in 1973 when Senator Jesse Helms amended a foreign aid bill. In 1999 Congress forced President Bill Clinton to accept a limited version of the gag rule in return for an agreement to pay the back dues the United States owed to the United Nations. Clinton instructed USAID officials to interpret the policy so as to minimize the impact on international family planning efforts and to respect the rights of citizens to speak freely on issues of importance to their countries (Rayman-Read 2001).

5. The Leipzig conference was itself part of the preparations for the FAO World Food Summit held in Rome 13–17 November 1996.

6. The text of the Leipzig Appeal can be found at http://navdanya.org/Templates/Templates/dwd/statement-leipzig.htm accessed 21 March 2007.

Chapter Three   The Triple Day: Women's Home, Community, and Workplace Environments

1. Schistosomiasis, filariasis, dengue, Chagas' disease, and leishmaniasis.

2. The role of biology in environmental health risk is related to endocrine disruptors, exogenous chemicals that mimic or antagonize the action of endogenous hormones in the human body. Research focuses on processes or tissues affected by estrogens, androgen blockers, and thyroid

hormones. Sex steroids affect the central nervous system, the immune system, and the reproductive system, while thyroid hormones affect most tissues in the human body (Sims and Butter 2000).

3. For a discussion of Vandana Shiva's work on food security see chapter 2.

4. In the 1908 case *Muller* v. *Oregon*, the U.S. Supreme Court upheld a law limiting the number of hours women could work each day because, the Court claimed, women are the guardians of the race and must protect their health, rather than because workers are entitled to occupational safety. These attitudes still prevailed at the end of the twentieth century. The Republic of Croatia seceded from Yugoslavia in 1990; its constitution prohibits night work for women in industry and protects mothers (maternity leave is generally 12 months); the law specifies work that women must not do, especially hard physical labor, work below ground, and work under water (Habitat 1995).

5. In recent U.K. documents, the five social classes are further refined in these eight categories: Higher managerial and professional occupations; lower managerial and professional occupations; intermediate occupations; small employers and own account workers; lower supervisory and technical occupations; semi-routine occupations; routine occupations; and long-term unemployed (including those who have never worked).

6. For a history of Korean legislation on maternity rights see http://www.kwdi.re.kr/data/02forum-1.pdf accessed 21 March 2007.

Chapter Four   Fighting for Good Health Services, Struggling with the Pharmaceutical Industry

1. Medact is a U.K.-based charity taking action on key global health issues such as the war on Iraq, collapsing health systems in Africa, and global climate change. WEMOS is a Dutch organization working with Southern partners on health issues including pharmaceutical supplies. The People's Health Movement (PHM) that has its roots deep in the grassroots people's movement calls for a revitalization of the principles of the Alma-Ata Declaration, which promised Health for All by the year 2000 and complete revision of international and domestic policy that has shown to impact negatively on health status and systems. The International People's Health Council (IPHC) is a worldwide coalition of people's health initiatives and socially progressive groups and movements committed to working for the health and rights of disadvantaged people—and ultimately of all people. IPHC is a founding member of the PHM and serves on the International Steering Committee of PHM.

2. Extensive documentation is available on the website of Human Rights Watch, Amnesty International, the American Friends Service Committee, Physicians for Human Rights, and the United Nations High Commission for Human Rights.

3. Health Action International (HAI), founded in 1981 to provide a voice for groups wanting to address the problems posed by the global pharmaceutical supply system, has grown into a regionalized informal network of over 200 autonomous network members in 70 countries.

4. The Coalition for the Medical Rights of Women (now called ACCESS) is a network of activists and health care professionals whose campaigns combine legal action, public policy development, self-help groups, and public education to create lasting changes in women's health care.

5. The Food and Drug Administration Modernization Act of 1997 (FDAMA Sec. 115 Clinical Investigations. (b) Women and Minorities) amended Section 505 (b) (1) 21 U.S.C. 355 (b) (1) mandated the review and development of guidance, as appropriate, on the inclusion of women in clinical trials. To implement this section, the agency formed the FDAMA women and minorities working group with representatives from the agency and the National Institutes of Health (FDA scholarship in women's health programs: participation of females in clinical trials and gender analysis of data in biologic product applications http://www.fda.gov/CbER/clinical/femclin.htm accessed 15 September 2006).

6. NitroMed, a US-based pharmaceutical company, has developed a new drug to treat heart failure specifically in African Americans, arguing that they have a higher rate of heart failure than the U.S. population as a whole and that they tend not to respond well to existing drugs (Pollack 2004).

7. A cross-sectional study is a descriptive study in which disease and exposure status are measured simultaneously in a given population. Cross-sectional studies provide a "snapshot" of the frequency and characteristics of a disease in a population at a particular point in time. A longitudinal study is a correlational research study that involves observations of the same items over long periods of time. Unlike cross-sectional studies, longitudinal studies track the same people, and therefore the differences observed in those people are less likely to be the result of cultural differences across generations (http://en.wikipedia.org/wiki/Main_Page accessed 15 September 2006).

8. The World Medical Association originally adopted the Declaration of Helsinki, Ethical Principles for Medical Research involving Human Subjects, in 1964 and amended it six times (in 1975, 1983, 1989, 1996, 2000, and 2002) (www.wma.net/e/policy/b.3htm accessed 10 July 2004).

9. Benatar and Singer (2000) complain of simplistic criticisms of clinical studies of HIV transmission during pregnancy; conditions in developed and developing countries are not comparable, they say, because pregnant women in developing countries attend antenatal clinics later than women in developed countries and are more often anemic and malnourished; thus the studies that established the efficacy of AZT in interrupting maternal-fetal transmission of the virus in developed countries were not necessarily applicable to women in developing countries. For another view see Rothman (2000).

10. For a nuanced account, more sympathetic to researchers, see Marks (2001).

Chapter Five The Sexual Politics of Violence against Women

1. Bellil died 4 September 2004, at age 31 of stomach cancer.

2. Until the later 1970s, similar laws existed in Italy and France and still exist in Spain and Portugal (Abu-Odeh 2000).

3. The Albadeel Coalition (2000) comprises Women to Women, the Feminist Center, the Crisis Center Hotline for Victims of Violence, the Center for the Aid of Sexually Abused Victims, Women Against Violence, Azl Siwar, the Arab Feminist Movement in Support of Victims of Sexual Abuse, the Arab Association of Human Rights, Al-Tufula Pedagogical Center, the Haifa Crisis Shelter, and the Democratic Women's Movement.

4. On 31 October 2006, Mukhtaran's memoir was released in the United States, titled *In the name of honor: a memoir.*

5. The 10 countries are Bangladesh, Botswana, Côte d'Ivoire, Ethiopia, Ghana, Honduras, Indonesia, Madagascar, Nepal, and Rwanda.

6. The countries that have banned FGC are Burkina Faso, Central African Republic, Chad, Côte d'Ivoire, Djibouti, Egypt, Ghana, Guinea, Senegal, Tanzania, and Togo. Nigeria has banned FGC under federal law, and in Kenya a presidential declaration has denounced the practice (Ben-Ari 2003).

7. The Coalition of Women for Peace is a regional network made up of 10 organizations, including Bat Shalom, Women in Black, the Israeli chapter of the Women's International League for Peace and Freedom, and Machsom-Watch, which monitors checkpoints for human rights violations. The coalition's main goal is to help end the occupation of Palestine through a peaceful resolution of the Israeli-Palestinian conflict. Member organizations lobby in cooperation on a wide range of issues, including equal involvement of women in peace negotiations, establishment of the state of Palestine alongside Israel based on 1967 borders and the recognition of Jerusalem as the shared capital of the two states. www.coalitionofwomen4peace.org.

8. Non-derogable prohibitions cannot be annulled or repealed.

Chapter Six   Women's Reproductive Rights

1. Latin American women's groups have rightly argued that if women cannot control their fertility and be free from sexual abuse and violence, they cannot function fully as responsible, participating members of families and communities: they cannot truly exercise citizenship. (author's note)

2. I base these observations on first-hand experience gained while working at WHO headquarters in the Maternal and Child Health Unit (MCH). Population control entered WHO in the 1960s with the creation of the Human Reproduction Unit, which emphasized research; by the 1970s family planning programs dominated MCH, and other units had to include family planning in their work to justify their budgets. This capture of programming extended to the other UN Specialized Agencies: ILO, FAO, UNESCO, and others all fell into line, incorporating family planning in their programs of work.

3. The Roman Catholic Church bases its position on the sanctity of life and is consistent in its opposition to birth control, abortion, the death penalty, and euthanasia. The Evangelical Christian churches do not base their opposition to birth control and abortion on the sanctity of life principle since they generally support the death penalty.

4. ICASC became the Women's Global Network for Reproductive Rights (WGNRR) with headquarters in Amsterdam.

5. UBINIG and Resistance Network (Bangladesh), Research Foundation for Science and Ecology (India), Third World Network (Malaysia), and People's Health Network (India), organized the Symposium on People's Perspectives on Population to consider issues of reproductive technologies and genetic engineering; they met in December 1993 in Comilla, Bangladesh, and issued the Comilla Declaration that outlines their strong opposition to population control and most modern reproductive technologies. One of the most articulate groups espousing this viewpoint is the Feminist International Network of Resistance to Reproductive and Generic Engineering (FINRRAGE), based in Germany.

6. The concept of citizenship relates to ideas of democracy and access to services but its meaning varies from place to place. In the United States, where immigrant rights are under attack, citizenship is a reactionary concept used to exclude aliens; in Latin America, women's groups use citizenship to involve the state in the needs and lives of people (WGNRR 1996c).

7. Protestant Britain permitted contraceptive advice in maternal and infant welfare clinics from 1930. The Catholic Church determined policies in Belgium, France, Portugal, Spain, and their colonies; women's movements in the metropolitan countries did not achieve change until the 1970s.

8. Redstockings was a radical feminist group founded in New York City in 1968; Susan Brownmiller (*Against our Will*) and Ellen Willis, a journalist, were members. CARASA (the Committee for Abortion Rights and Against Sterilization Abuse) organized in New York City in 1976; it grew out of protest against the Hyde Amendment to Title XIX of the Social Security Act that ended federal Medicaid payments for abortion (Nelson 2003).

9. In 2004 Health Watch UP Bihar and Ramakant Rai took their case against the federal government of India to the Indian Supreme Court; the case alleged coercion and abusive practices resulting from poor quality of care in government-run sterilization camps and failure to comply with national guidelines on the performance of sterilization that establish mandatory procedures for obtaining informed consent. In March 2005, the Supreme Court ordered state governments to take immediate steps to regulate health care providers who perform sterilization procedures and to compensate women who suffer complications due to sub-standard practices and the relatives of victims who may die from botched operations (Center for Reproductive Rights www.crlp.org accessed 30 July 2006).

10. NB: where abortions are illegal, accurate statistics on deaths are lacking and probably politicized.

11. In Uruguay, at the Pereira Rossel Hospital, unsafe abortions caused 47 percent of maternal deaths from 1996 to 2001 in women between 19 and 45 years of age (WGNRR 2003e).

12. Eighteen countries participated: Argentina, Australia, Bangladesh, Brazil, Ethiopia, Fiji, France, Guyana, India, Ireland, Italy, Kenya, Lithuania, Mexico, Nigeria, Poland, South Africa, and the United States. All but Argentina, Ethiopia, Fiji, France, Ireland, Lithuania, and Nigeria contributed case studies to the final publication.

13. Doctors inject hormones to stimulate the donor's ovaries to release large numbers of eggs, followed by frequent blood tests and ultrasound scans to determine the timing of retrieval; the procedure entails insertion of a needle in the ovaries to aspirate the eggs.

14. According to Surrogate Parenting Services, Inc. the approximate cost is $61,250 (http://www.surrogateparenting.com/financial.asp, accessed 10 July 2006); Circle Surrogacy quotes a cost of between $38,560 to $52,410 (http://www.circlesurrogacy.com/costs.html, accessed 10 July 2006).

15. In January 2004 the agency reversed its decision, permitting saline implants only and deferring approval; it asked Inamed for more studies and more information. FDA voiced concerns about implants that rupture or leak without knowing the consequences. The agency wanted to know how women could determine if their device failed and asked whether women should have frequent magnetic resonance imaging tests (MRIs) to look for silicone implant ruptures (Kolata 2004b).

Chapter Seven   Toward a New Universalism

1. Universal design is an inclusive approach to design that enables as many people as possible regardless of age, ability, or situation to use products, services, and environments.

2. Among the Indian groups represented were All India Federation of the Deaf; Action for Ability Development and Inclusion (AADI) (formerly The Spastics Society of Northern India); National Federation of the Blind; and the National Trust for the Welfare of People with Autism, Cerebral Palsy and Mental Retardation.

3. The term social inclusion was first used in France by René Lenoir, former Secrétaire d'État à l'Action Sociale in the publication, *Les exclus: un français sur dix* in 1974. The British picked up social exclusion in the 1980s, using it somewhat differently to refer to hierarchies of power. In the United States, where the term is not common, social exclusion is written about in concepts of the underclass, discrimination, and disadvantage.

4. Rousseau viewed society as a cooperative community, postulating a cultural and moral social bond between the individual and society. This paradigm of solidarity implies the nation's responsibility to individuals, not just the government's responsibility but also that of all members of society. Rousseau claimed that the state of nature eventually degenerates into a brutish condition without law or morality, at which point the human race must adopt institutions of law or perish. In the degenerate phase of the state of nature, man is prone to compete frequently with other men while at the same time becoming increasingly dependent on them. This double pressure threatens both his survival and his freedom. By joining together through the social contract and abandoning their claims of natural right, individuals can both preserve themselves and remain free. Rousseau believed that submission to the authority of the general will of the people as a whole guarantees individuals against being subordinated to the will of others and also ensures their obedience because they are, collectively, the authors of the law.

5. Thomas Hobbes' competitive social order and view of human life—that it is nasty, brutish, and short—are by now clichés; he believed that interest groups compete for survival and power. His paradigm is one of individual responsibility. In later versions of this view, political philosophers like John Locke (1632–1704) believed in democracy and in a social contract that holds a society

of competitive individualists together. By social contract Locke meant an agreement on basic values and normative arrangements. Social and economic failures are understood to be personal or familial (Krieger 2001).

6. Weber's monopoly paradigm emphasizes hierarchical power relations in the constitution of social order. Group monopolies are responsible for exclusion, since powerful groups restrict the access of outsiders through social closure. Inequality overlaps with such group distinctions, but social democratic citizenship and participation in the community mitigate inequality (de Haan 2001).

7. The human development index (HDI) measures longevity, education, and standard of living. The gender development index (GDI) measures gender disparities in basic human capabilities, and the human poverty index (HPI) reflects the percentage of people who suffer from deprivation relating to survival, knowledge, and a decent standard of living. All of the measures focus on national averages, not on specific groups, and on outcomes rather than on the actors and processes that cause them (de Haan 1998).

8. Human security means safety from chronic threats like hunger, disease, and repression; it includes job security, income security, environmental security, and security from crime. It also means protection from sudden and hurtful disruptions in the patterns of daily life (UNDP 1994).

9. Paper presented at the seminar on "Macro-Meso-Micro Social Influences in Health: Changing Patterns of Morbidity and Mortality" organized by the International Union for the Scientific Study of Population (IUSSP) and held in Yaoundé, Cameroon, 5–8 June 2002.

BIBLIOGRAPHY

Abd El Hadi, A. 2000. Female genital mutilation in Egypt. In *African women's health* edited by M. Turshen, 145–166. Trenton: Africa World Press.

Abdullah, R. 2003. NGO advocacy on women's health and rights in Southeast Asia. *Development* 46(2):33–37.

Abraham, M. 2000. *Speaking the unspeakable: marital violence among South Asian immigrants in the United States*. New Brunswick: Rutgers University Press.

Abu-Odeh, L. 2000. Crimes of honor and the construction of gender in Arab societies. In *Women and sexuality in Muslim societies* edited by P. Ilkkaracan, 363–380. Istanbul, Turkey: Women for Women's Human Rights.

Abusharaf, R.M. and A.M. Abdel Halim. 2000. Female circumcision, the case of Sudan. In *African women's health* edited by M. Turshen, 125–143. Trenton: Africa World Press.

Adekanye, T.O. 1999. Women's reproductive health and food growing/processing: the case of Nigeria. Paper prepared for the regional workshop on Women's Reproductive Health and Household Food Security in Rural Africa organized by the Economic Commission for Africa Food Security and Sustainable Development Division. Addis Ababa: Economic Commission for Africa.

Akeroyd, A.V. 2004. Coercion, constraints, and "cultural entrapments": a further look at gendered and occupational factors pertinent to the transmission of HIV in Africa. In *HIV & AIDS in Africa: beyond epidemiology* edited by E. Kalipeni, S. Craddock, J.R. Oppong, and J. Ghosh, 89–103. Oxford: Blackwell Publishing.

Akinrimisi, A. 2003. *Women's Global Network for Reproductive Rights Newsletter* 78(1):17–21.

Alam, N., S.K. Saha, and J.K. van Ginneken. 2000. Determinants of divorce in a traditional Muslim community in Bangladesh. Max-Planck-Gesellschaft http://www.demographic-research.org/Volumes/Vol3/4 accessed 8 August 2006.

Albadeel Coalition. 2000. Albadeel Coalition against family honor crimes. In *Women and sexuality in Muslim societies* edited by P. Ilkkaracan, 399–402. Istanbul, Turkey: Women for Women's Human Rights.

Al-Dawla, A.S. 2000. The story of the FGM taskforce: an ongoing campaign against female genital mutilation. In *Women and sexuality in Muslim societies* edited by P. Ilkkaracan, 427–433. Istanbul, Turkey: Women for Women's Human Rights.

Ali, A.H. 2006. Women go "missing" by the millions. *International Herald Tribune* 25 March.

Amin, S. 1995. Fifty years is enough! *Monthly Review* April:8–50.

Amnesty International. 1998. Women's rights in South Korea. London: AI Index: ASA 25/20/98.

Amnesty International. 1999. United States of America. Rights for all. Not part of my sentence. Violations of the human rights of women in custody. London: AI Index: AMR 51/019/1999.

Amnesty International. 2001. Medical concern. Torture and ill-treatment of women in pre-trial detention, Lebanon. London: AI Index: MDE 18/014/2001.

———. 2005. Annual report. www.amnesty.org accessed 21 July 2005.

Anderson, P. 2005. The family world system. *The Nation* 30 May.

Angell, M. 2004. The truth about the drug companies. *New York Review of Books* LI(12):52–58.

Antrobus, P. 2004. *The global women's movement: origins, issues and strategies.* London: Zed Books.

ARROW. 2001. Women's health and rights in Southeast Asia: a Beijing monitoring report. Kuala Lumpur: The Asia-Pacific Resource and Research Center for Women.

Arsu, S. 2005. Turks to fight "honor killings" of women. *The New York Times* 16 May.

Association Démocratique des Femmes du Maroc. 2003. NGOs' report on the implementation of the CEDAW Convention: a parallel report to the periodic report of the Government of Morocco. Presented to the United Nations Committee on the Elimination of Discrimination Against Women (CEDAW). www.mediterraneas.org/IMG/pdf/cdaw-Maroc.pdf accessed 1 April 2007.

Astbury, J. 2002. Mental health: gender bias, social position, and depression. In *Engendering international health: the challenge of equity* edited by G. Sen, A. George, and P. Östlin, 143–168. Cambridge, MA: MIT Press.

Auyero, J. and T.P. Moran. 2007. The dynamics of collective violence: dissecting food riots in contemporary Argentina. www.socialresearch.newschool-edu/centers/haney/conf04-Javier-Auyero.pdf accessed 1 April 2007.

Avotri, J.Y. and V. Walters. 1999. You just look at our work and see if you have any freedom on earth: Ghanaian women's accounts of their work and their health. *Social Science & Medicine* 48:1123–1133.

AWID. 2005. Where is the money for women's rights? Assessing resources and the role of donors in the promotion of women's rights and the support of women's rights organizations. The Association for Women's Rights in Development, www.awid.org accessed 26 March 2007.

Bacon, D. 2005. Stories from the borderlands. *NACLA* 39(1):25–30.

Badran, M. 1995. *Feminists, Islam, and nation: gender and the making of modern Egypt.* Princeton: Princeton University Press.

Bala Nath, M. 2000. Women's health and HIV: experiences from a sex workers' project in Calcutta. *Gender and Development* 8(1):100–108. www.ids.ac.uk/blds/ejournals/ej-list.html accessed 26 March 2007.

Bandarage, A. 1997. *Women, population and global crisis: A political-economic analysis.* London: Zed Books.

Banerji, D. 1992. Family planning in the nineties: more of the same or a sharp break? *Economic and Political Weekly* XXVII(17).

Bard, J.S. 2002. Unjust rules for insanity. *New York Times* 13 March.

Barker, P. 1991. *Regeneration,* London: Viking.

Barrig, M. 1994. The difficult equilibrium between bread and roses: women's organizations and democracy in Peru. In *The women's movement in Latin America. Participation and democracy* edited by Jane Jaquette, 151–175. Boulder: Westview Press.

———. 1999. The persistence of memory: feminism and the state in Peru in the 1990s. Ford Foundation Civil Society and Democratic Governance in the Andes and the Southern Cone Comparative Regional Project. PUCP Department of Social Sciences.

Barthelemy, F. 2004. Peru: the scandal of forced sterilization. *Le Monde Diplomatique* May:8–9.

Baumgardner, J. 2002. When in Rome. . . . *The Nation* 2 December:22–24.

Beall, J., O. Crankshaw, and S. Parnell. 2002. *Uniting a divided city: governance and social exclusion in Johannesburg.* London: Earthscan Publications.

Bearak, B. 2000. Women are defaced by acid and Bengali society is torn. *New York Times* 24 June:A1.

Beleoken, E. 2003. Cameroonian Committee of Reflection on Abortion (CCRA). *Women's Global Network for Reproductive Rights Newsletter* 78(1):10.

Bellil, S. 2002. *Dans l'enfer des tournantes*. Paris: Denoël.

Bellows, A.C. 2003. Exposing violences: using women's human rights theory to reconceptualize food rights. *Journal of Agricultural and Environmental Ethics* 16:249–279.

Ben-Ari, N. 2003. Villagers join campaigns against female genital mutilation. *Women's Global Network for Reproductive Rights Newsletter* 78(1):28–29.

Benatar, S. and P. Singer. 2000. A new look at international research ethics. *BMJ* 321:824–826.

Bennett, O. 1990. *Panos dossier: triple jeopardy: women and AIDS*, London: Panos Institute. www. aegis.com/pubs/panos/1990/TripleJeopardy_Women_and_AIDS.asp accessed 26 March 2007.

Bennett, S., J.D. Quick, and G. Velasquez. 1997. Public-private roles in the pharmaceutical sector: implications for equitable access and rational drug use. Geneva: World Health Organization.

Bennis, P. 1990. *From stones to statehood: the Palestinian uprising*. New York: Olive Branch Press.

Benson, J.E. 1994. The effects of packinghouse work on Southeast Asian refugee families. In *Newcomers in the workplace: immigrants and the restructuring of the U.S. economy* edited by L. Lamphere, A. Stepick, and G. Grenier, 99–126. Philadelphia: Temple University Press.

Berer, M. 2002. Making abortions safe: a matter of good public health policy and practice. *Reproductive Health Matters* 10(19):31–42.

Bernstein, N. and L. Kaufman. 2004. Women likelier to be slain by a partner than a stranger. *New York Times* 22 October.

Bhalla, N. 2005. India wakes up to its battered women. *Reuters* 5 July.

Bhattacharyya, S. 2003. Quinacrine sterilization (QS): the ethical issues. *International Journal of Gynecology and Obstetrics* 83 Suppl.2:S13–S21.

Bhutta, Z., S. Nundy, and K. Abbasi. 2004. Editorial: is there hope for South Asia? Yes, if we can replicate the models of Kerala and Sri Lanka. *BMJ* 328:777–778, 3 April.

Bickenbach, J.E., S. Chatterji, E.M. Bradley, and T.B. Üstün. 1999. Models of disablement, universalism and the international classification of impairments, disabilities and handicaps. *Social Science & Medicine* 48:1173–1187.

Black, E. 2003. *War against the weak: eugenics and America's campaign to create a master race*. New York: Four Walls Eight Windows.

Bodenheimer, T. 2000. Uneasy alliance—clinical investigators and the pharmaceutical industry. *New England Journal of Medicine* 342:1539–1544.

Bonner, R. 2003a. A challenge in India snarls foreign adoptions. *New York Times* 23 June:A3.

———. 2003b. For poor families, selling baby girls was economic boon. *New York Times* 23 June:A3.

Bossen, L. Missing girls, land, and population controls in rural China. www.cicred.org/Eng/Seminars/Details/Seminars/FDA/FDdraftpapers.htm accessed 27 March 2007.

Breines, I., R. Connell and I. Eide, eds. 2000. *Male roles, masculinities and violence: a culture of peace perspective*. Paris: UNESCO.

Breton, M.J. 1998. *Women pioneers for the environment*. Boston: Northeastern University Press.

Broadway, M. 1994. Beef stew: cattle, immigrants and established residents in a Kansas beefpacking town. In *Newcomers in the workplace: immigrants and the restructuring of the U.S. economy* edited by L. Lamphere, A. Stepick, and G. Grenier, 25–43. Philadelphia: Temple University Press.

Brockerhoff, M. and P. Hewitt. 2000. Inequality of child mortality among ethnic groups in sub-Saharan Africa. *Bulletin of the World Health Organization* 78(1):30–41.

Brody, J. 2000. Exposing the perils of eating disorders. *New York Times* 12 December.

Brown, H. 2006. One spoonful at a time. Sunday *New York Times* Magazine 17 December.

Burdon, R. 2003. *The suffering gene—environmental threats to our health*. London: Zed Books.

Burt, J.-M. 1998. Sterilization and its discontents. *NACLA Report on the Americas* 31(5), March–April.

Butalia, U. 1997. The women's movement in India: action and reflection. *Communique* 42–43, July–August. www.twnside.orgsg/title/India-cn.htm accessed 27 March 2007.

Butcher, K. and A. Welbourn. 2001. Danger and opportunity: responding to HIV with vision. *Gender and Development* 9(2):51–61. www.ids.ac.uk/blds/ejournals/ej-list.html accessed 26 March 2007.

Butterfield, F. 2002. Wife killings at fort reflect growing problem in military. *New York Times* 29 July:A9.

Caldwell, J., P. Caldwell, and P. Quiggan. 1989. Disaster in an alternative civilization: the social dimensions of AIDS in Sub-Saharan Africa. Canberra: National Centre for Epidemiology and Population Health.

Campbell, B. 2000. New rules of the game: the World Bank's role in the construction of new normative frameworks for states, markets and social exclusion. *Canadian Journal of Development Studies* XXI(1):7–30.

Canadian Women's Committee on Population and Development. 1996. Bill of rights for contraceptive research, development and use. Ottawa: Canadian Women's Committee.

Carapico, S. 2000. NGOs, INGOs, GO-NGOs, and DO-NGOs: making sense of non-governmental organizations. *Middle East Report* 214:12–15.

Caton, A. 2002. Fighting CRACKDown. *Resist* 11(8):3.

Cerón, A., A. Das, and M. Fort. 2004. The struggle for people's health. In *Sickness and health: the corporate assault on global health* edited by M. Fort, M.A. Mercer, and O. Gish, 161–166. Cambridge, MA: South End Press.

Chambers, R. 1989. Vulnerability: how the poor cope. *IDS Bulletin* 20(2).

Charkiewicz, E. 2004. Beyond good and evil: notes on global feminist advocacy. *Women in Action* 2 August:50. www.isiswomen.org/wia/wia2-04/ewa.htm accessed 1 April 2007.

Chavkin, W. 2003. Chipping away at Roe. *The Nation* 30 June:24.

Chesler, E. 2001. New options, new politics. *The American Prospect* Fall:A12–A14.

Chesler, P.1972. *Women and madness.* New York: Doubleday.

Chu, H. 2006. Wombs for rent, cheap. *The Los Angeles Times* 19 April.

Commission on Human Rights. 2005. Report of the Special Rapporteur on the right of everyone to the enjoyment of the highest attainable standard of physical and mental health, Paul Hunt. Addendum: Summary of cases transmitted to governments and replies received. E/CN.4/2005/51/Add.1, 2 February.

———. 2006. Report of the Special Rapporteur on the right of everyone to the enjoyment of the highest attainable standard of physical and mental health, Paul Hunt. New York: United Nations E/CN.4/2006/48, 3 March.

Commission on Macroeconomics and Health. 2001. Macroeconomics and health: investing in health for economic development. Geneva: World Health Organization.

Connell, D. 2001. *Rethinking revolution: new strategies for democracy and social justice.* Lawrenceville, NJ: Red Sea Press.

Coomaraswamy, R. 1998. Report of the Special Rapporteur on violence against women, its causes and consequences. UN Commission on Human Rights Fifty-fourth session E/CN.4/1998/54.

———. 2001. Contribution on the subject of race, gender and violence against women. World Conference against Racism, Racial Discrimination, Xenophobia and Related Intolerance. A/CONF.189/PC.3/5 27 July.

Cooper, C. 2002. A cancer grows. *The Nation* 6 May:30–34.

Cordell, D.D., J.W. Gregory, and V. Piché. 1987. African historical demography: The search for a theoretical framework. In *African Population and Capitalism: Historical Perspectives* edited by D.D. Cordell and J.W. Gregory, 12–32. Boulder: Westview Press; republished Madison: University of Wisconsin Press, 1994.

Coulibaly, S.O. and M. Keita. 1993. Les comptes nationaux de la santé au Mali: 1988–1991. New York: United Nations Children's Fund (UNICEF), l'initiative de Bamako rapport technique numéro 18, juillet.

Craddock, S. 2004. AIDS and ethics: clinical trials, pharmaceuticals, and global scientific practice. In *HIV and AIDS in Africa: beyond epidemiology* edited by E. Kalipeni, S. Craddock, J.R. Oppong, and J. Ghosh, 240–251. Oxford: Blackwell Publishing.

CRLP. 2006. Abortion laws fact sheet. Center for Reproductive Law and Policy. www.reproductiverights.org/pub_fac_abortion_laws.html. accessed 27 March 2007.

CWPE. 1995. Statement on women, population and environment: call for a new approach. *Political Environments* Summer Issue, 2:40. Hampshire College: Committee on Women, Population and the Environment.

DABINDU Collective. 1999/2000. A report on the situation of women workers in the free trade zones of Sri Lanka. *Women's Global Network for Reproductive Rights Newsletter* 68/69(4/1):7–10.

Daines, V. and D. Seddon. 1993. Confronting austerity: women's responses to economic reform. In *Women's lives and public policy: the international experience* edited by M. Turshen and B. Holcomb, 3–32. Westport, CT: Praeger.

Das, V. 1995. National honor and practical kinship: unwanted women and children. In *Conceiving the new world order: the global politics of reproduction* edited by F.D. Ginsburg and R. Rapp, 212–233. Berkeley: University of California Press.

de Gruchy, J. and S. Lewin. 2001. Ethics that exclude: the role of ethics committees in lesbian and gay health research in South Africa. *American Journal of Public Health* 91(6):865–868.

de Haan, A. 1998. Social exclusion: an alternative concept for the study of deprivation? *IDS Bulletin* 29(1):10–18.

———. 2001. Social exclusion: enriching the understanding of deprivation. www.sussex.ac.uk/Units/SPT/journa/archive/pdf/issue2-2.pdf accessed 27 March 2007.

de Haan, A. and S. Maxwell. 1998. Editorial: poverty and social exclusion in North and South. *IDS Bulletin* 29(1), January.

De Koninck, M. 1998. Reflections on the transfer of "progress": the case of reproduction. In *The politics of women's health: exploring agency and autonomy* edited by S. Sherwin, 150–177. Philadelphia: Temple University Press.

Decosas, J. 2002. The social ecology of AIDS in Africa. Geneva: United Nations Research Institute for Social Development.

Desjarlais, R., L. Eisenberg, B. Good, and A. Kleinman, eds. 1995. Women. In *World mental health: problems and priorities in low-income countries* edited by R. Desjarlais, L. Eisenberg, B. Good, and A. Kleinman, 179–206. New York: Oxford University Press.

Dixon, B. 2001. Exclusive societies: towards a critical criminology of post-apartheid South Africa. *Society in Transition* 32(2): 205–227.

DSM IV. 1994. Diagnostic and statistical manual of mental disorders. Washington, DC: American Psychiatric Association.

Dugger, C.W. 2000. Kerosene, weapon of choice for attacks on wives in India. *New York Times* 26 December:A1.

———. 2001. Modern Asia's anomaly: the girls who don't get born. *New York Times* 6 May.

Dunkle, K.L., R. Jewkes, H. Brown, G. Gray, J. McIntyre, and S. Harlow. 2004. Gender-based violence, relationship power, and risk of HIV infection in women attending antenatal clinics in South Africa. *Lancet* 363:1415–1421.

Düzkan, A. and F. Koçali. 2000. An honor killing: she fled, her throat was cut. In *Women and sexuality in Muslim societies* edited by P. Ilkkaracan, 381–387. Istanbul, Turkey: Women for Women's Human Rights.

Edelman, H.S. 1994. Why is Dolly crying? *Journal of Popular Culture* Winter: 19–32.

Editorial. 2005. The Women of Gitmo. *New York Times* 15 July.

Ekeh, P. 1975. Colonialism and the two publics in Africa: a theoretical statement. *Comparative Studies in Society and History* 17:91–112.

El Saadawi, Nawal. 1999. *A daughter of Isis: the autobiography of Nawal El Saadawi.* London: Zed Books.

El-Gawhary, K.M. 2000. Egyptian advocacy NGOs: catalysts for social and political change? *Middle East Report* Spring, 214:38–41.

Elliston, J. 2003. Eugenics in North Carolina: thousands were sterilized by the state. *Southern Exposure* Spring:11–12.

Elliston, J. and C. Lutz. 2003. Hidden casualties. *Southern Exposure* Spring:25–31.

Epstein, H. 2004. The fidelity fix. *New York Times Magazine* 13 June.

Epstein, S. 1991. Democratic science? AIDS activism and the contested construction of knowledge. *Socialist Review* 21(2):35–64.

———. 1994. Women at risk are still in the dark. *The Los Angeles Times* 9 September.

———. 1994. Environmental pollutants as unrecognized causes of breast cancer. *International Journal of Health Services* 24(1):145–150.

———. 1997. Awareness month keeps women perilously unaware. *The Chicago Tribune* 27 October.

Epstein, S. and S. Rennie. 1992. Perspectives on medicine: a travesty at women's expense. *The Los Angeles Times* 22 June.

ERA/FoEN. 2002. http://acas.prairienet.org/bulletin/bull68toc.html accessed 27 March 2007.

Eschle, C. and N. Stammers. 2004. Taking part: social movements, INGOs, and global change. *Alternatives: Global, Local, Political* June–July, 29(3):333

European Commission. 2005. The situation of Roma in an enlarged European Union. Luxembourg: Office for Official Publications of the European Communities.

Everett, J.M. 1979. *Women and social change in India.* New York: St Martin's Press.

Farha, L. 2000. Contextualizing violence against women: forced evictions in situations of armed conflict. *Canadian Woman Studies* 19(4):71–76.

Faucett, J. 1997. The ergonomics of women's work. In *Women's health: complexities and differences* edited by S.B. Ruzek, V.L. Olesen, and A.E. Clarke, 154–171. Columbus: Ohio University Press.

Ferguson, S. 2001. Boom or bust. *Mother Jones* May/June:30.

Fikree, F.F. and O. Pasha. 2004. Role of gender in health disparity: the South Asian context. *BMJ* 328:823–826, 3 April.

Fisher, I. 2002. Account of Punjab rape tells of a brutal society. *New York Times* 17 July.

Fix, M. and L. Laglagaron. 2002. Social Rights and Citizenship: An International Comparison. Washington: DC: The Urban Institute. www.urban.org/UploadedPDF/410545-SocialRights.pdf accessed 27 March 2007.

Fonn, S. 2004. Getting cervical screening onto the agenda. Johannesburg: Women's Health Project. www.wits.ac.za/whp/cancer.htm accessed 8 August 2006.

French, H.W. 2003. Victims say Japan ignores sex crimes committed by teachers. *New York Times* 29 June:A4.

Fuller, T. 2006. A vision of pale beauty carries risks for Asia's women. *New York Times* 14 May.

Gabriel, T. 1996. High tech pregnancies test hope's limit. *New York Times* 7 January:A1, 18, 19.

Gakidou, E.E., C.J.L. Murray, and J. Frenck. 2000. Defining and measuring health inequality: an approach based on the distribution of health expectancy. *Bulletin of the World Health Organization* 78(1):42–54.

Gall, C. 2001. Macedonia village is center of Europe web in sex trade. *New York Times* 28 July:A1.

———. 2004. For more Afghan women, immolation is escape. *New York Times* 8 March.

Garcia-Moreno, C. and A. Claro. 1994. Population and ethics: expanding the moral space. In *Population Policies Reconsidered* edited by G. Sen, L.C. Chen, and A. Germaine, 15–26. Boston: Harvard School of Public Health. http://www.hsph.harvard.edu/rt21/globalism/ CLARO.html accessed 15 June 2006.

Garcia-Moreno, C., C. Watts, H. Jansen, M. Ellsberg, and L. Heise. 2003. Responding to violence against women: WHO's multicountry study on women's health and domestic violence. *Health and Human Rights* 6(2):113–127.

Gardner, J. and J. El Bushra, eds. 2004. *Somalia—the untold story: the war through the eyes of Somali women.* London: CIIR and Pluto Press.

Geiger, H.J. 2002. Racial and ethnic disparities in diagnosis and treatment: a review of the evidence and a consideration of the causes. In *Unequal Treatment: Confronting Racial and Ethnic Disparities,* edited by B.D. Smedley, A.Y. Smith, and A.R. Nelson, 216–247. Washington, DC: National Academy of Sciences.

George, R. 2003. Revolt against the rapists. *The Guardian* 5 April. www.guardian.co.uk accessed 10 November 2004.

———. 2004. Samira Bellil: courageous writer who forced France to confront the outrage of gang rape. *The Guardian* 13 September. www.guardian.co.uk accessed 10 November 2004.

Germain, A., K.K. Holmes, P. Piot, and J.N. Wasserheit, eds. 1992. *Reproductive tract infections: global impact and priorities for women's reproductive health.* New York: Plenum Press.

Giller, J. 1998. Caring for "victims of torture" in Uganda: some personal reflections. In *Rethinking the trauma of war* edited by P.J. Bracken and C. Petty. London/New York: Free Association Books.

Glenn, David. 2004. A dangerous surplus of sons? *The Chronicle of Higher Education* 50(34):A14, April 30.

Global Health Watch. 2005. *Global health watch, 2005–2006: an alternative world health report.* London: Zed Books.

Global Rights. 2004. Economic position of women: Bosnia and Herzegovina NGO shadow report to the UN CEDAW Committee. Washington, DC. www.globalrights.org accessed 30 July 2005.

Goldberger, N.R., N. Goldberger, and B. Clinchey, eds. 1996. *Knowledge, difference, and power: essays inspired by women's ways of knowing.* New York: Basic Books.

Golden, F. 1998. Boy? Girl? Up to you. *Time* 21 September:82–83.

Goosen, M. and B. Klugman, eds. 1996. *The South African women's health book.* Cape Town: Oxford University Press.

Gordon, L. 1977. *Woman's body, woman's right.* Harmondsworth: Penguin Books.

Gore, C. 1994. Social exclusion and Africa south of the Sahara: a review of the literature. IILS Discussion Paper. Geneva: International Institute of Labour Studies.

Grady, D. 2003. Women with genetic mutation at high risk for breast cancer, study confirms. *New York Times* 24 October.

Green, P.S. 2003a. Gypsies in Slovakia complain of sterilizations. *New York Times* 28 February.

———. 2003b. A rocky Polish landfall for a Dutch abortion boat. *New York Times* 24 June.

Greenhouse, L. 2000. Should a fetus's well-being override a mother's rights? *New York Times* 9 September.

Grimes, D.A. 2003. Unsafe abortion: the silent scourge. *British Medical Bulletin* 67:99–113.

Guenena, N. and N. Wassef. 1999. *Unfulfilled promises: women's rights in Egypt.* www.popcouncil.org/pdfs/unfulfilled_promises.pdf accessed 27 March 2007.

Güezmes García, A. 1999/2000. Women's reproductive rights in Peru. *Women's Global Network for Reproductive Rights Newsletter* 68/69(4/1):46–47.

Gungaloo, R. 2003. 33,000 letters asking men to act responsibly. *Women's Global Network for Reproductive Rights Newsletter* 78(1):32–33.

Gupta, A.S. 1999. Infrastructure development in health care and the pharmaceutical industry: implications of the World Development Report 1993. In *Disinvesting in health: the World Bank's prescriptions for health* edited by M. Rao, 143–162. New Delhi: Sage Publications.

Gupta, G.R. and E. Weiss. 1993. Women's lives and sex: implications for AIDS prevention culture. *Medicine and Psychiatry* 17(4): 399–412.

Gwatkin, D.R. 2002. Reducing health inequalities in developing countries. www.worldbank.org accessed 3 August 2005.

Habitat. 1995. Report of the international workshop on women's access, control and tenure of land, property and settlement. Gävle, Sweden: United Nations.

Hammami, R. 2000. Palestinian NGOs since Oslo: from NGO politics to social movements. *Middle East Report* Spring, 214:16

Harcourt, W. 2003. Editorial: the reproductive health and rights agenda under attack. *Development* 46(2):3–5.

————. 2006. The global women's rights movement: power politics around the United Nations and the World Social Forum. Geneva: UNRISD Programme on Civil Society and Social Movements number 25.

Hartmann, B. 1995. *Reproductive rights and wrongs: the global politics of population control.* Cambridge: South End Press.

————. 1997. Population control in the new world order. In *Development for Health*, edited by D. Eade, 80–85. Oxford: Oxfam Publishing.

————. 2001. Sterilization abuse escalates in India. *The Fight for Reproductive Freedom* XVI(1):8.

Hartocollis, A. 2006. Nearly 8 years later, guilty plea in subway killing. *New York Times* 11 October.

Harvard School of Public Health. *The global burden of disease and injury series.* www.hsph.harvard.edu/Organizations/bdu/GBDseries.html accessed 27 March 2007.

Hatem, M.F. 1994. The paradoxes of state feminism in Egypt. In *Women and Politics Worldwide* edited by B.J. Nelson and N. Chowdhury, 226–242. New Haven: Yale University Press.

————. 2000. The professionalization of health and the control of women's bodies as modern governmentalities in nineteenth century Egypt. In *Women and sexuality in Muslim societies* edited by P. Ilkkaracan, 67–79. Istanbul, Turkey: Women for Women's Human Rights.

Henwood, D. 2000. Indicators: health and wealth. *The Nation* 10 July:10.

Hermans, M. 2005. Challenges in connecting the global and the local levels. *Women's Global Network for Reproductive Rights Newsletter* 86(3):5–7.

Heyzer, N. 2001. Leadership for human security to create a world free of violence. www.unifem.undp.org/speaks/GAthirdcom2001.html.Hlatshwayo, Z. and B. Klugman. 2001. A sexual rights approach. *Agenda* 47:14–20.

Hochschild, A.R. 2000. The nanny chain. *The American Prospect* 3 January: 32–36.

Hodgson, D. and S. Cotts Watkins. 1997. Feminists and neo-Malthusians: past and present alliances. *Population and Development Review* 23(4):469–523.

Hoge, W. 2005. U.N. charges Sudan ignores rapes in Darfur by military and police. *New York Times* 30 July.

Hollingshead, A.B. and F.C. Redlich. 1958. *Social class and mental illness.* New York: Wiley.

Hoosain, M., R. Jewkes, and S. Maphumalo. 1998. *MRC Newsletter.* South Africa.

HRG. 1997. Letter to the Department of HHS concerning their funding of unethical trials which administer placebos to HIV-infected pregnant women through NIH and the Centers for Disease Control. (HRG Publication #1415) http://www.citizen.org/publications/release.cfm?ID=6612 accessed 27 March 2007.

HRW. 1993a. *Human rights watch world report 1994.* Washington, DC: Human Rights Watch.

————. 1993b. A modern form of slavery: trafficking of Burmese women and girls into brothels in Thailand. Washington, DC: Human Rights Watch.

————. 1996. No guarantees: sex discrimination in Mexico's maquiladora sector. New York: Human Rights Watch.

————. 2004. Trafficking in women and girls in Bosnia and Herzegovina. New York: Human Rights Watch.

————. 2005. Darfur: women raped even after seeking refuge. New York: Human Rights Watch.

————. 2006. Swept under the rug: abuses against domestic workers around the world. New York: Human Rights Watch.

Huggler, J. 2006. First doctor jailed over India's aborted girls. *The Independent* (UK) 30 March.

ICTR. 1998. *The prosecutor vs Jean-Paul Akayesu*, Case No. ICTR-96-4-T, decision of 2 September 1998, para. 731. United Nations International Criminal Tribunal on Rwanda.

Inhorn, M.C. 2003. Global infertility and the globalization of new reproductive technologies: Illustrations from Egypt. *Social Science & Medicine* 56:1837–1851.

International Women's Health Coalition. 2004. Peru. http://www.iwhc.org/programs/latin_america/peru/colleagues.cfm accessed 12 June 2006.

Iyer A. and G. Sen. 2000. Health sector changes and health equity in the 1990s in India. In *Health and equity* edited by S. Roghuram. Bangalore: HIVOS, technical report series 1.8.

Jeeves, A.H. and O.J.M. Kalinga. 2002. *Communities at the margin: studies in rural society and migration in southern Africa, 1890–1980*. Pretoria: University of South Africa.

Jesani, A., N. Madwidalla, and M. Gupte. 2001. Pre-natal diagnostic techniques in India: a crisis of credibility. *Women's Global Network for Reproductive Rights Newsletter* 74(3):16–17.

Jewkes, R. 2002. Intimate partner violence: causes and prevention. *Lancet* 359:1423–1429.

Jiang, Q., M.W. Feldman, X. Jin. 2005. Estimation of the number of missing females in China: 1900–2000. Paper presented at the International Union for the Scientific Study of Population XXV International Population Conference, Tours, France, 18–23 July 2005. www.iussp2005.princeton.edu/abstractVierwer.aspx?submissionId=51345 accessed 8 August 2006.

Jok, J. M. 1999. Militarism, gender and reproductive suffering: the case of abortion in Western Dinka. *Africa/International African Institute* 69(2): 194–212.

Kabeer, N. 1996. Agency, well-being and inequality: reflections on the gender dimensions of poverty. *IDS Bulletin* 27 (1).

Kafka, B. 2003. Disability rights vs. workers rights: a different perspective. Znet November 14. http://www.zmag.org/content/print_article.cfm?itemID=4503&sectionID=47 accessed 4 January 2007.

Kaplan, L. 1996. *The story of Jane, the legendary underground feminist abortion service*. New York: Pantheon Books.

Karides, M. 2002. Linking local efforts with global struggles: Trinidad's National Union of Domestic Employees. In *Women's activism and globalization: linking local struggles and transnational politics* edited by N.A. Naples and M. Desai, 156–171. New York: Routledge.

Kark, S. and E. Kark. 1999. *Promoting community health: from Pholela to Jerusalem*. Johannesburg: Witwatersrand University Press (available from Africa Book Centre info@africabookcentre.com).

Kay, B., A. Germain, and M. Bangser. 1991. The Bangladesh Women's Health Coalition. *Quality* 3, 1991. www.popcouncil.org/pdfs/qcq/qcq03.pdf accessed 27 March 2007.

Key, S.W. and M. Marble. 1996. Market for women's pharmaceuticals reaches $5.7 billion in 1995. *Cancer Biotechnology Weekly* 4 March:14–16.

Kimbrell, A. 1993. *The human body shop: the engineering and marketing of life*. San Francisco: HarperSanFrancisco.

Kishwar, M. 2002. *Off the beaten track: rethinking gender justice for Indian women*. New Delhi: Oxford University Press.

Kisseka, M.N. 1990. Gender and mental health in Africa. *Women Therapy* 10(3):1–13.

Kligman, G. 1995. Political demography: the banning of abortion in Ceausescu's Romania. In *Conceiving the new world order: the global politics of reproduction* edited by F. D. Ginsburg and R. Rapp, 234–255. Berkeley: University of California Press.

Klugman, B. 1994. Feminist methodology in relation to the Women's Health Project. In *Gender, health, and sustainable development*, edited by P. Wijeyaratnew, L.J. Arsenault, J.H. Roberts, and J. Kitts, 187–202. Lanham, MD: Bernan Press.

Koehler, C.S.W. 2006. Pharmaceuticals for all: The story of WHO and the "essential drugs." *thetimeline* http://pubs.acs.org/subscribe/journals/mdd/v04/i06/html/06timeline.html accessed 15 September 2006.

Koerner, B.I. 2002. Disorders made to order. *Mother Jones* July/August:58–81.

Kolata, G. 2000. Without fanfare, morning-after pill gets a closer look. *New York Times* 8 October.

———. 2004a. The heart's desire. *New York Times* 11 May.

———. 2004b. F.D.A. defers final decision about implants. *New York Times* 9 January.

———. 2006. Hormones and cancer: assessing the risks. *New York Times* 26 December.

Krieger, J. 2001. *The Oxford companion to politics of the world.* Oxford: Oxford University Press. Second edition.

Kuczynski, A. 2006. Beauty junkies: inside our $15 billion obsession with cosmetic surgery. New York: Doubleday.

Kumar, R. 1995. From Chipko to Sati: the contemporary Indian women's movement. In *The challenge of local feminisms: women's movements in global perspective* edited by A. Basu, 58–86. Boulder, CO: Westview Press.

Kushner, R. 1975. *Breast cancer: A personal history and investigative report.* New York: Harcourt Brace Jovanovich.

Lawrence, J. 2000. The Indian Health Service and the sterilization of Native American women. *The American Indian Quarterly* 24(3):400–419.

Lerner, B.H. 2001. *The breast cancer wars: hope, fear, and the pursuit of a cure in 20ᵗʰ century America.* New York: Oxford University Press.

Lerner, S. 1996. The price of eggs: undercover in the infertility industry. *Ms* March/April:28–34.

Levy, C. 2002a. For mentally ill, death and misery. *New York Times* 28 April.

———. 2002b. Here, life is squalor and chaos. *New York Times* 29 April.

———. 2002c. Voiceless, defenseless and a source of cash. *New York Times* 30 April.

———. 2002d. Ingredients of a failing system: a lack of state money, a group without a voice. *New York Times* 28 April.

Lewontin, R. 2000. *The triple helix: gene, organism, and environment.* Cambridge: Harvard University Press.

Limanowska, B. 2001. Employed by the global sex industry. *Women's Global Network for Reproductive Rights Newsletter* 73(2):14–15.

Lobe, E. 2002. Violence against women: the case of Cameroon. *Women's Global Network for Reproductive Rights Newsletter* 77(3):35–36.

Lohmann, L. 2003. Re-imagining the population debate. The Corner House briefing 28. www.thecornerhouse.org.uk accessed 27 March 2007.

Lorde, A. 1994. Living with cancer. In *The black women's health book* edited by E.C. White, 27–37. Seattle: Seal Press.

Louie, M.C.Y. 2001. *Sweatshop warriors: immigrant women workers take on the global factory.* Cambridge, MA: South End Press.

Lumsden, M.A. 2005. The hormone replacement therapy controversy. *BJOG: an International Journal of Obstetrics and Gynaecology* 112: 689–691.

Lutz, C. and J. Elliston. 2002. When several soldiers killed their wives, an old problem was suddenly news. *The Nation* 275(12):18–21.

Lyall, S. 2002. Lost in Sweden: a Kurdish daughter is sacrificed. *New York Times* 23 July.

Mackintosh, M. 2003. Health care commercialisation and the embedding of inequality. Geneva: UNRISD. www.unrisd.org accessed 27 March 2007.

MacLean, J. 1980. Roots of the women's movement. *Socialist Review* 50–51:233–243.

Madunagu, E. 2001. Nigeria: why adolescents avoid health centers. *Women's Global Network for Reproductive Rights Newsletter* 74(3):15.

Malhotra, R. 2001. The politics of the disability rights movements. *New Politics* 8(3).

Mamdani, M. 1996. *Citizen and subject: contemporary Africa and the legacy of late colonialism.* Princeton: Princeton University Press.

Manchester, J. and P. Mthembu. 2002. Positive women: voices and choices. *Brief* 11. Brighton, U.K.: Institute of Development Studies/ BRIDGE.

Manjate, R., R. Chapman, and J. Cliff. 2000. Lovers, hookers, and wives: unbraiding the social contradictions of urban Mozambican women's sexual and economic lives. In *African Women's Health* edited by M. Turshen. Trenton: Africa World Press.

Markel, H. 2003. The ghost of medical atrocities: what's next, after the unveiling? *New York Times* 23 December.

Marks, J. 2003. Against the genetic grain. *The Nation* 7 April:29–31.

Marks, L. 2001. *Sexual chemistry: a history of the contraceptive pill.* New Haven: Yale University Press.

Marris, V. 1996. May I be a mother? Disabled women and motherhood. *Women's Global Network for Reproductive Rights Newsletter* 54:23–24.

Martin, E. 1994. *Flexible bodies.* Boston: Beacon.

McNeil, D.G. 2006. In raising the world's I.Q., the secret's in the salt. *New York Times* 16 December.

Meier, B. 2004a. A.M.A. urges disclosure on drug trials. *New York Times* 16 June.

———. 2004b. A medical journal quandary: how to report on drug trials. *New York Times* 21 June.

Meintjes, S., A. Pillay and M. Turshen, eds. 2002. *The aftermath: women in post-conflict transformation.* London: Zed Books,

Melrose, D. 1982. *Bitter pills: medicines and the Third World poor.* Oxford: OXFAM.

Mensch, B.S., J. Bruce, and M.E. Greene. 1998. *The unchartered passage: girls' adolescence in the developing world.* New York: The Population Council.

Messing, K. and S. de Grosbois. 2001. Women workers confront one-eyed science: building alliances to improve women's occupational health. *Women & Health* 33(1/2):125–141.

Michaels, W.B. 2006. The trouble with diversity. *American Prospect* 12 September:18–22.

Mintz, M. 1965. *The therapeutic nightmare.* Boston: Houghton Mifflin.

Mogollón, M.E. 1999/2000. Nothing personal—the practice of surgical contraception in Peru. *Women's Global Network for Reproductive Rights Newsletter* 68/69(4/1):45–46.

Molyneux, M. and S. Razavi. 2006. Beijing plus 10: an ambivalent record on gender justice. United Nations Research Institute for Social Development Occasional Paper 15.

Morgen, S. 2002. *Into our own hands: the women's health movement in the United States, 1969–1990.* New Brunswick: Rutgers University Press.

Morsy, S.A. 1995. Deadly reproduction among Egyptian women: maternal mortality and the medicalization of population control. In *Conceiving the new world order: the global politics of reproduction* edited by F.D. Ginsburg and R. Rapp, 162–176. Berkeley: University of California Press.

Moser, C. and F. Clarke, eds. 2001. *Victors, perpetrators or actors: gender, armed conflict and political violence.* London: Zed Books.

Movimiento Manuela Ramos (Manuela Ramos Movement) http://www.civil-society.oas.org/accredited%20organizations/Movimiento%20Manuela%20Ramos%20-%20CPCISC-16305/CP14048E08.doc accessed 25 June 2006.

Ms. 1996. Beauty and the breast. March/April:45–57.

———. 1997. Peruvian women challenge an ugly rape law. March/April:18.

Mthembu, P. 1998. A positive view. *Agenda* 39:26–29.

Mumbai, R.S. 2001. India: women's groups protest at new contraceptive trial. *Women's Global Network for Reproductive Rights Newsletter* 74(3):22–23.

Murray, C.J.L., R. Govindaraj, and G. Chellaraj. 1994. Global domestic expenditures in health. Washington, DC: The World Bank, Background Paper No. 13.

Muthengi, A. 2003. Kenyan widows fight wife inheritance. 18 November. http://news.bbc.co.uk/ 1/hi/world/africa/3275451.stm accessed 27 March 2007.

Mydans, S. 2001. Sexual violence as tool of war: pattern emerging in East Timor. *New York Times* 1 March.

Napoli, M. 1996. Look back in anger. *Ms.* May/June: 40–42.

Narrigan, D. et al. 1997. Research to improve women's health. In *Women's health: complexities and differences* edited by S.B. Ruzek, V.L. Olesen, and A.E. Clarke, 551–579. Columbus: Ohio State University Press.

Nathan, D. 1999. Work, sex and danger in Ciudad Juárez. *NACLA* XXXIII (3):24–30.

Nduna, S. and D. Rude. 1998. A safe space created by and for women. New York: International Rescue Committee, March.

Nelson, J. 2003. *Women of color and the reproductive rights movement.* New York: New York University Press.

NGOs in Bosnia and Herzegovina. 2004. Shadow report on the implementation of CEDAW and women's human rights in Bosnia and Herzegovina. Presented to the United Nations Committee on the Elimination of Discrimination Against Women (CEDAW).

Norsigian, J.D., V. Diskin, P. Doress-Worters., J. Pincus, W. Sanford, and N. Swenson. 2002. The Boston Women's Health Book Collective and Our Bodies, Ourselves: a brief history and reflection. *Women's Health Journal* 72, April. www.ourbodiesourselves.org/about/jamwa.asp accessed 27 March 2007.

Notman, M.T. and Nadelson, C. 2002. The hormone replacement therapy controversy. *Archives of Women's Mental Health* 5:33–35.

Nottingham, W.J. 2004. Lori Berenson's Story. October 25, http://www.counterpunch.org/ nottingham10252004.html.

Off Road Pakistan. 2005. http://ko.offroadpakistan.com/pakistan/2004_10/mukhtaran_bibi_ sentenced_to_be_raped.html accessed 26 July 2005.

Ogu, C. and L.R. Wolfe.1994. Midlife and older women and HIV/AIDS. Washington, DC: Center for Women Policy Studies.

Ojiambo Ochieng, R. 2003. Supporting women and girls' sexual and reproductive health and rights: the Ugandan experience. *Development* 46(2):38–44.

Omvedt, G. 1993. *Reinventing revolution: new social movements and the socialist tradition in India.* London: M.E. Sharpe.

Onori, A. 2006. *Intellectual property and access to medicines.* Geneva: Centrale Suisse Romande.

Östlin, P. 2002. Examining work and its effects on health. In *Engendering international health: the challenge of equity* edited by G. Sen, A. George and P. Östlin, 63–81. Cambridge, MA: MIT Press.

Oxaal, Z. with S. Cook. 1998. Health and poverty gender analysis. Brighton: Institute of Development Studies, University of Sussex, BRIDGE Report No 46.

Padilla, Beatriz. 2004. Grassroots participation and feminist gender identities: a case study of women from the popular sector in metropolitan Lima, Peru. *Journal of International Women's Studies* 6(1):93–113.

PAHO. 2005. Gender equality policy. Washington, DC: Pan American Health Organization.

PANOS. 1998. The intimate enemy: gender violence and reproductive health. London: Briefing No. 27.

———. 2002. Patents, pills and public health: can TRIPS deliver? London: The PANOS Institute.

———. 2003. Beyond victims and villains: addressing sexual violence in the education sector. London: The Panos Institute.

Paolisso, M. and J. Leslie. 1995. Meeting the changing health needs of women in developing countries. *Social Science and Medicine* 40(1):56–65.

Parker, R. and P. Aggleton. 2003. HIV and AIDS-related stigma and discrimination: a conceptual framework and implication for action. *Social Science and Medicine* 57:13–24.

Patierno, C. 1997. With child. In *The lesbian health book* edited by J. White and M.C. Martinez, 181–188. Seattle: Seal Press.

Petchesky, R.P. 2003. *Global prescriptions: gendering health and human rights*. London: Zed Books.

Petchesky, R.P. and K. Judd, eds. 1998. *Negotiating reproductive rights: women's perspectives across countries and cultures*. London: Zed Books.

Pichardo, N.A. 1997. New social movements: a critical review. *Annual Review of Sociology* Annual 23:411.

Pies, C. 1997. The ongoing politics of contraception. In *Women's health: complexities and differences* edited by S.B. Ruzek, V.L. Olesen, and A.E. Clarke. 520–546. Columbus: Ohio State University Press.

Pilipina. 1995. Building sisterhood in the Filipino women's movement. *Women's Global Network for Reproductive Rights Newsletter* 50:10–12.

Pollack, A. 2004. Drug approved for heart failure in black patients. *New York Times* 20 July.

Qadeer, I. 1998. Reproductive health—a public health perspective. *Women's Global Network for Reproductive Rights Newsletter* 64(4):20–25.

Quisumbing, A.R., L. Haddad, and C. Peña. 2001. Are women overrepresented among the poor? An analysis of poverty in ten developing countries. Washington, DC: International Food Policy Research Institute.

Ragged Edge Online. 2003. The eugenics apologies. www.ragged-edge-mag.com/1103/1103ft1.html accessed 3 August 2005.

Rao, M. 1997. Quinacrine "trials" and the national security questions in the USA. *Women's Global Network for Reproductive Rights Newsletter* 57(1):7.

——. 1999. The structural adjustment programme of the *World Development Report 1993*: implications for family planning in India. In *Disinvesting in health: the World Bank's prescription for health* edited by Mohan Rao, 80–106. New Delhi: Sage Publications.

——. 2005. India's population policies: untouched by the Cairo rhetoric. *Development* 48(4):21–27.

Rapp, R. 1999. Testing women, testing the fetus: the social impact of amniocentesis in America. New York, London: Routledge.

Rayman-Read, A. 2001. The sound of silence. *The American Prospect* Fall:A21–A24.

Richardson, L. and A. Kirsten. 2005. Armed violence and poverty in Brazil: a case study of Rio de Janeiro and assessment of Viva Rio for the armed violence and poverty initiative. University of Bradford Center for International Cooperation and Security. www.brad.ac.uk/acad/cics/publications/AVPI/poverty/AVPI_Rio_de_Janeiro.pdf accessed 27 March 2007.

Richmond, A.H. 2002. Social exclusion: belonging and not belonging in the world system. *Refuge: Canada's Periodical on Refugees* 21(1):40–48.

Ritchie, B.E. 1996. *Compelled to crime: the gender entrapment of battered black women*. London: Routledge.

Rizvi, H. 2006. United Nations: treaty shines light on disabled inequality. IPS, New York, 13 December.

Rizvi, Z. 2004. Mukhtaran Bibi: sentenced to be raped. http://ko.offroadpakistan.com/pakistan/2004_10/mukhtaran_bibi_sentenced_to_be_raped.html accessed 26 July 2005.

Roberts, D. 1997. *Killing the black body: race, reproduction and the meaning of liberty*. New York: Pantheon Books.

Rodgers, G. 1997. Labour-market exclusions and the role of social actors. In *Social exclusion and antipoverty policy: a debate* edited by C. Gore and J. Figueiredo. International Institute of Labour Studies, Geneva.

Rogo, K.O., D.R. Gwatkin, J.F. May, A.E. Elmendorf, M. Rani, and A. Soucat. 2002. Health, nutrition, and population equity and outcomes in Sub-Saharan Africa: implications for HNP strategies and engagement of African researchers. World Bank, unpublished paper.

Rohter, L. 2007. In the land of bold beauty, a trusted mirror cracks. *New York Times* 14 January.

Roth, R. 2000. *Making women pay: the hidden costs of fetal rights*. Ithaca: Cornell University Press.

Rothman, D. 2000. The shame of medical research. *The New York Review of Books* XLVII(19):60–64.

Rousseau, S. 2006. Women's citizenship and neopopulism: Peru under the Fujimori regime. *Latin American Politics and Society* 48(1): 117–141.

Ruggi, S. 2000. Commodifying honor in female sexuality: honor killings in Palestine. In *Women and sexuality in Muslim societies* edited by P. Ilkkaracan, 393–398. Istanbul, Turkey: Women for Women's Human Rights.

Rutherford, C. 1992. Reproductive freedoms and African American women. *Yale Journal of Law and Feminism* 4(2):255–290.

Ruzek, S. 1986. Feminist vision of health: an international perspective. In *What is feminism* edited by J. Mitchell and A. Oakley, 184–207. NY: Pantheon.

Ruzek, S.B. and J. Becker. 1999. The women's health movement in the United States: from grass-roots activism to professional agendas. *Journal of the American Medical Women's Association* 54:4–8.

Ruzek, S.B., V.L. Olesen, and A.E. Clarke. 1997. What is women's health? In *Women's health: complexities and differences* edited by S.B. Ruzek, V.L. Olesen, and A.E. Clarke, 1–28. Columbus: Ohio State University Press.

Safa, H.I. 1986. Runaway shops and female employment: the search for cheap labor. In *Women's work: development and the division of labor by gender* edited by E. Leacock and H.I. Safa, 58–71. New York: Bergin & Garvey.

Sai, F. 2004. International commitments and guidance on unsafe abortion. *African Journal of Reproductive Health* 8(1):15–28.

Salzinger, L. 2001. Making fantasies real: producing women and men on the maquila shop floor. *NACLA* March:13–19.

Sample, I. 2006. Drug firms accused of turning healthy people into patients. *The Guardian* UK 11 April.

Sarwar, B. 2002. Brutality cloaked as tradition. *New York Times* 6 August:A15.

Sawhney, A. 1999. Women's empowerment and health experiences from Rajasthan. In *Disinvesting in health: the World Bank's prescriptions for health* edited by M. Rao, 172–182. New Delhi: Sage Publications.

Scarpaci, J. 1993. Empowerment strategies of poor urban women under the Chilean dictatorship. In *Women's lives and public policy: the international experience* edited by M. Turshen and B. Holcomb, 33–50. Westport: Greenwood Press.

Schuler, M. 1992. Violence against women: an international perspective. In *Freedom from violence: women's strategies from around the world* edited by M. Schuler, 1–45. NY: UNIFEM.

Scott, A. M. 1990. Patterns of patriarchy in the Peruvian working class. In *Women, employment and the family in the international division of labour* edited by S. Stichter and J.L. Parpart, 198–220. Philadelphia: Temple University Press.

Seaman, B. 1995. *The doctors' case against the pill*. Alameda, CA: Hunter House, 25th anniversary edition.

Sen, A. 1999. *Development as freedom*. New York: Anchor Books.

———. 2000. Population and gender equity. *The Nation* July 24/21:16–18.

Sen, G., A. George, and P. Östlin. 2002. Engendering health equity: a review of research and policy. Cambridge: Harvard Center for Population and Development Studies Working Paper Series 12(2).

SEWA. 2000. Workshop at World Water Forum. The Hague.

Sharma, R. 2000. AIDS vaccine research focuses on subtypes in developed world. *BMJ* 321(7264):787.

Sideris, T. 2003. War, gender and culture: Mozambican women refugees. *Social Science & Medicine* 56:713–724.

Sidibé, K.A. 1999/2000. The practice of female circumcision in Mali. *Women's Global Network for Reproductive Rights Newsletter* 68/69(4/1):49–50.

Silliman, J., M.G. Fried, L. Ross, and E. Gutiérrez. 2004. *Undivided rights: women of color organize for reproductive justice*. Cambridge: South End Press.

Sims, J. and M.E. Butter. 2000. Gender equity and environmental health. Cambridge, MA: Harvard Center for Population and Development Studies Working Paper Series 10(6).

Sjöström, H. and R. Nilsson. 1972. *Thalidomide and the power of the drug companies*. Harmondsworth: Penguin Books.

Snow, C.P. 1993. *The two cultures*. Cambridge: Cambridge University Press.

Soares, V., A.A.A. Costa, C.M. Buarque, D.D. Dora, and W. Sant'anna. 1995. Brazilian feminists and women's movements: a two-way street. In *The challenge of local feminisms: women's movements in global perspective* edited by A. Basu, 302–323. Boulder: Westview Press.

Solinger, R. 2002. *Beggars and choosers: how the politics of choice shapes adoption, abortion, and welfare in the United States*. New York: Hill & Wang.

Som, R. 1994. Jawaharlal Nehru and the Hindu Code: a victory of symbol over substance? *Modern Asian Studies* 28(1):165–194.

Sorenson, D. 1997. *The invisible victims*. Washington, DC: U.S. Department of Education, Office of Educational Research and Improvement, Educational Resources Information Center.

Sow, F. and C. Bop. 2004. *Notre corps, notre santé: la santé et la sexualité des femmes en Afrique subsaharienne*. Paris: L'Harmattan.

Sparr, P. ed. 1994. *Mortgaging women's lives: feminist critiques of structural adjustment*. London: Zed Books.

Stein, D. 2002. Reproductive rights are labor rights. *Resist* 11(8).

Stemerding, B. 1997. International women's health meeting. *Women's Global Network for Reproductive Rights Newsletter* 58(2):4.

Stevens, P.E. 1998. The experiences of lesbians of color in health care encounters. In *Gateways to improving lesbian health and health care* edited by C.M. Ponticelli, 77–93. New York: Haworth Press.

Stull, D.D. 1994. Knock 'em dead: work on the killfloor of a modern beefpacking plant. In *Newcomers in the workplace: immigrants and the restructuring of the U.S. economy* edited by L. Lamphere, A. Stepick, and G. Grenier, 44–77. Philadelphia: Temple University Press.

Sudanese Feminist Union. 1996. The feminist movement in Sudan. In *The feminist movement in the Arab world* edited by the New Woman Research and Study Center, 59–81. Giza, Egypt: New Woman Research and Study Center.

Sundari Ravindran, T.K. 1997a. Biology and destiny. *Reproductive Health Matters* November:18–28.

———. 1997b. Research on women's health: some methodological issues. *Development for Health*, Oxfam, 14–22.

Sussman, M.B. 1969. Readjustment and rehabilitation of patients. In *Poverty and health: a sociological analysis* edited by J. Kosa, A. Antonovsky, and I.K. Zola, 244–264. Cambridge: Harvard University Press.

Svirsky, G. 2004. License to kill. www.coalitionofwomen.org accessed 27 November 2004.

Swarup, H.L., N. Sinha, C. Ghosh, and P. Rajput. 1994. Women's political engagement in India: some critical issues. In *Women and politics worldwide* edited by B. J. Nelson and N. Chowdhury, 361–379. New Haven: Yale University Press.

Sweetman. C. 1997. Magda Mateus Cardenas Director of Centro Amauta, Cusco, Peru. *Gender and Development* 5(1):62–66.

Tabengwa, M. 2003. *HIV/AIDS and the world of work.* Gaborone: BONELA.

Taipale, I., ed. 2002. *War or health? A reader.* London: Zed Books.

Tallis, V. 2002. *Gender and HIV/AIDS: overview report.* Brighton, U.K.: University of Sussex IDS/Bridge.

Tantiwiramanond, D. and S.R. Pandey. 1991. *By women, for women: a study of women's organizations in Thailand.* Singapore: Institute of Southeast Asian Studies.

Tarkan, L. 2002. Fertility clinics begin to address mental health. *New York Times* 8 October.

Tarlo, E. 2000. Body and space in a time of crisis: sterilization and resettlement during the emergency in Delhi. In *Violence and Subjectivity* edited by V. Das, A. Kleinman, M. Rampele, and P. Reynolds, 242–270. Berkeley, CA: University of California Press.

The Corner House and WGNRR. 2004. A decade after Cairo: women's health in a free market economy. www.thecornerhouse.org.uk./briefing/index.shtml accessed 20 June 2006.

The Lancet. 2004. WHO argues the economic case for tackling violence 363:2058, 19 June www.thelancet.com accessed 29 July 2005.

The New Woman Research and Study Center. 1996. *The feminist movement in the Arab world.* Giza, Egypt: The New Woman Research and Study Center.

Therborn, G. 2004. *Between sex and power: family in the world, 1900–2000.* London and New York: Routledge.

Tipping, G. and M. Segall.1995. Health care seeking behaviour in developing countries. Brighton, U.K.: Institute of Development Studies, Development Bibliography 12.

Townsend, P. and N. Davidson. 1982. *The Black report: inequalities in health.* Harmondsworth: Penguin Books.

Turshen, M. 1975. *The political economy of health, with a case study of Tanzania.* Brighton, U.K.: University of Sussex unpublished doctoral thesis.

———. 1995. Societal instability in international perspective: relevance to HIV/AIDS prevention. Workshop on the Social and Behavioral Science Base for HIV/AIDS Prevention and Intervention, National Academy of Sciences, Washington, DC, 12 June.

———. 1999. *Privatizing Health Services in Africa.* New Brunswick: Rutgers University Press.

———. 2004. Definitions and injuries of violence. In *Interventions: activists and academics respond to violence* edited by E.A. Castelli and J.R. Jakobsen, 29–35. New York: Palgrave.

Turshen, M. and O. Alidou. 2000. Africa: women in the aftermath of civil war. *Race & Class* 41(4):81–92.

U.K. Office for National Statistics. 2004. *Focus on social inequalities.* http://www.statistics. gov.uk/ STATBASE/Product.asp?vlnk=13488 accessed 16 January 2006.

Uganda Bureau of Statistics. 2002. Census data available from P.O. Box 13, Entebbe, Uganda. E-mail: ubos@infocom.co.ug.

UN. 1996. *Platform for action and the Beijing Declaration.* New York: UN Department of Public Information.

———. 2000a. United Nations releases most recent statistics on world's women. New York: UN Press release 31 May.

———. 2000b. The world's women: trends and statistics. New York: United Nations.

———. 2004. Interim report submitted by the Special Rapporteur of the Commission on Human Rights on torture and other cruel, inhuman or degrading treatment or punishment. A/59/324.

———. 2005 Social and economic situation of Palestinian women 1990–2004. New York: United Nations E/ESCWA/WOM/2005/Technical Paper.1.

UNAIDS. 2002. Impact of AIDS on older populations. www.unaids.org accessed 27 March 2007.

———. 2006. 2006 report on the global AIDS epidemic. New York: UNAIDS.

UN Commission on Human Rights. 1994. Sub-Commission on Prevention of Discrimination and Protection of Minorities. Report of the second United Nations Regional Seminar on

Traditional Practices Affecting the Health of Women and Children. E/CN.4/Sub.2/1994/10 28 July 1994.

UNDESA. 2003. World contraceptive use. United Nations Department of Economic and Social Affairs Population Division.

UNDP. 1994. *Human development report 1994*. New York: Oxford University Press.

———. 2000. *Human development report 2000*. New York: Oxford University Press.

———. 2004. *Human development report 2004*. New York: Oxford University Press.

UN Forward-Looking Strategies for the Advancement of Women. 1985. http://www.un.org/esa/gopher-data/conf/fwcw/nfls/nfls.en accessed 3 January 2007.

UNHCR. 2005. Woman forced to carry fatally impaired fetus to term wins case. New York, November 17. http://www.reproductiverights.org/pr_05_1117KarenPeru.html accessed 30 July 2006.

UN High Commissioner for Human Rights Sub-commission on Human Rights. Traditional practices affecting the health of women and the girl child. Resolution 2000/10. (CN.4/2001/2—E/CN.4/Sub.2/2000/46).

UNICEF. 2005. *The state of the world's children 2005*. www.unicef.org accessed 10 August 2005.

UNIFEM. 2005. Gender profile of the conflict in Timor-Leste. www.womenwarpeace.org accessed 30 July 2005.

United Nations Press Release. 2001. Committee experts note difficulties for Nicaragua in efforts to improve situation of women. http://www.un.org/News/Press/docs/2001/wom1296.doc.htm accessed 1 June 2006.

UNRISD. 2000. Visible hands—taking responsibility for social development. Geneva: United Nations Research Institute for Social Development.

———. 2006 Gender equality: striving for justice in an unequal world. Geneva: United Nations Research Institute for Social Development.

Vargas, V. and V. Villanueva. 1994. Between confusion and the law: women and politics in Peru. In *Women and politics worldwide* edited by B.J. Nelson and N. Chowdhury, 575–589. New Haven: Yale University Press.

Vatz, R.E. 2006. Those crazy insanity pleas. *USA Today Magazine* September.

Vetten, L. and K. Bhana. 2001. Violence, vengeance and gender: a preliminary investigation into the links between violence against women and HIV/AIDS in South Africa. *Research Report*. Johannesburg and Cape Town: Centre for the Study of Violence and Reconciliation. Available from info@csvr.org.za.

Wagstaff, A. 2000. Socioeconomic inequalities in child mortality: comparisons across nine developing countries. *Bulletin of the World Health Organization* 78(1):19–29.

Waitzkin, H. 2003. Report on macroeconomics and health: a summary and critique. *The Lancet* 361:526, February 8. www.thelancet.com accessed 11 August 2005.

Waldman, A. 2003. States in India take new steps to limit births. *New York Times* 7 November.

Wallace, D. and R. Wallace, 1998. *A plague on your houses: how New York was burned down and national public health crumbled*. London, New York: Verso.

Wang, I.-S. 2002. Results and issues of the labour laws-related women reform movements. *Women's Global Network for Reproductive Rights Newsletter* 76(2):15–17.

Waters, H., A. Hyder, Y. Rajkotia, S. Basu, and J.A. Rehwinkel. 2004. *The economic dimensions of interpersonal violence*. Geneva: World Health Organization.

Webb, G. 1996. The dark alliance. *San Jose Mercury News* 22 August.

WEDO. 1992. Women's action agenda 21. http://www.iisd.org/women/action21.htm accessed 27 June 2006.

Westley, S.B. 1995. Evidence mounts for sex-selective abortion in Asia. *Asia-Pacific Population and Policy* May/June, no.34:1–4.

WGNNR. 1999/2000. The ousting of sex workers in Tanbazar, Bangladesh. *Women's Global Network for Reproductive Rights Newsletter* 68/69:50–51.

WGNRR. 1995. Poor women's health remains poor: a critique of the Beijing document. *Women's Global Network for Reproductive Rights Newsletter* 50:12–14.

———. 1996b. Canada gets tough with reproductive technologies. *Women's Global Network for Reproductive Rights Newsletter* 55/56:21.

———. 1996c. International members meeting: a report of discussion. *Women's Global Network for Reproductive Rights Newsletter* 55/56:1–24.

———. 1997. Enforced chastity in Lombok, Indonesia? *Women's Global Network for Reproductive Rights Newsletter* 57(1):11.

———. 2000. Health for all women, health for all now! *Women's Global Network for Reproductive Rights Newsletter* 4(1): 2–5.

———. 2000a. I am not a virus, I am a strong voice, listen to me. *Women's Global Network for Reproductive Rights Newsletter* 71(3):16–17.

———. 2000b. Rwanda: women demonstrate against violence. *Women's Global Network for Reproductive Rights Newsletter* 71(3):19.

———. 2000c. The new global gag rule: a violation of democratic principles and international human rights. *Women's Global Network for Reproductive Rights Newsletter* 71(3):20–21.

———. 2001a. Women's health and environments network in Canada. *Women's Global Network for Reproductive Rights Newsletter* 73(2):29–30.

———. 2001b. Tamil Nadu campaign against sex selective abortion. *Women's Global Network for Reproductive Rights Newsletter* 73(2):32.

———. 2002a. International trade agreements and women's access to healthcare. Amsterdam: Women's Global Network for Reproductive Rights.

———. 2002b. Quinacrine alert network. *Women's Global Network for Reproductive Rights Newsletter* 76(2):24–25.

———. 2002c. Governor apologises for forced sterilizations. *Women's Global Network for Reproductive Rights Newsletter* 76(2):24.

———. 2002c. Quinacrine sterilizations are advertised and offered in Florida. *Women's Global Network for Reproductive Rights Newsletter* 76(2):24.

———. 2002d. A study on women's experiences with Depo Provera. *Women's Global Network for Reproductive Rights Newsletter* 77(3):42–43.

———. 2002e. Which comes first, the woman or the egg? Women protest ban of emergency contraceptive pill. *Women's Global Network for Reproductive Rights Newsletter* 77(3):43–44.

———. 2003a. Evaluation of the anti-fertility vaccine campaign (1993–2001). *Women's Global Network for Reproductive Rights Newsletter* 78(1):5.

———. 2003b. Vatican says word "gender" is anti-church code. *Women's Global Network for Reproductive Rights Newsletter* 78(1):42.

———. 2003c. Pakistan: 520 women gang raped during the year 2002. *Women's Global Network for Reproductive Rights Newsletter* 78(1):42–43.

———. 2003d. Parents pay to choose baby's sex. *Women's Global Network for Reproductive Rights Newsletter* 78(1):43.

———. 2003e. Declaration in preparation of the international day of action for women's health. *Women's Global Network for Reproductive Rights Newsletter* 78(1):39.

———. 2003f. Women say "no" to the privatization of primary health center. *Women's Global Network for Reproductive Rights Newsletter* 78(1):38.

———. 2003g. Serbia and Montenegro: women create peace: less armaments, more health and knowledge. *Women's Global Network for Reproductive Rights Newsletter* 78(1):36–38.

Whitehead, M., G. Dahlgren, and T. Evans. 2001. Equity and health sector reforms: can low-income countries escape the medical poverty trap? *Lancet* 358: 833–836.

Whittaker, A. 2003. Abortion law reform advocacy in Thailand. *development* 46(2):72–79.

WHO. 1999. An assessment of reproductive health needs in Ethiopia. WHO/RHR/HRP/ITT/99.1.

WHO. 2000a. *World health report 2000*. Geneva: World Health Organization.

———. 2000b. Gender, health and poverty. Geneva: WHO Fact Sheet #251, June.

———. 2000c. Women, ageing and health. Fact sheet #252, June.

———. 2001. Mental health: strengthening mental health promotion. Fact sheet #220.

———. 2002b. Towards a common language for functioning, disability and health: ICF. Geneva: World Health Organization.

———. 2002a. *Weekly Epidemiological Record* 20, 17 May.

———. 2003a. *WHO pharmaceuticals newsletter* 3.

———. 2003b. Assisted reproduction in developing countries—facing up to the issues. *Progress in Reproductive Health Research* no. 63.WHO. 2004. WHO-UNICEF Joint Statement on Anaemia. http://www.who.int/topics/anaemia/en/who_unicef-anaemiastatement.pdf accessed 27 March 2007.

———. 2006. Female genital mutilation and obstetric outcome: WHO collaborative prospective study in six African countries. *Lancet* 367:1835–1841.

Wilson, E. 2007. Health guidelines suggested for models. *New York Times* 6 January.

Winerip, M. 1999. Report faults care of man who pushed woman onto tracks. *New York Times* 5 November.

Wingard, D.L. 1993. Patterns and puzzles. In *Women's health: complexities and differences* edited by S.B. Ruzek, V.L. Olesen, and A.E. Clarke, 29–45. Columbus: Ohio State University Press.

Wolf, N. 1990. *The beauty myth*. London: Chatto and Windus.

Women's Health Action Foundation. 1995. *A healthy balance? Women and pharmaceuticals*. www.haiweb.org accessed 15 September 2006.

Women's Health Project. 2001. Advocating for abortion access: eleven country studies. Johannesburg: Witwatersrand University Press.

Women's Health Project Newsletter. 1992. www.wits.ac.za/whp/newsletter.htm accessed 27 March 2007.

Women's Net. http://www.apc.org/intersections/issue1.shtml?x=287 accessed 26 June 2006.

Women's Rights Project and Americas Watch. 1993. *Untold terror: violence against women in Peru's armed conflict*. Human Rights Watch.

Women's Rights Project and Middle East Watch. 1992. Punishing the victim: rape and mistreatment of Asian maids in Kuwait. New York: Human Rights Watch.

Worcester, N. and M.H. Whatley. 2000. More selling of HRT: still playing on the fear factor. In *Women's health* edited by N. Worcester and M.H. Whatley, 317–335. Dubuque: Kendall/Hunt Publishing

World Bank. 1993. *World development report 1993*. Oxford: Oxford University Press.

———. 1997. *World development report 1997*. Oxford: Oxford University Press.

———. 2003. Global poverty goals within reach. News Release 2003/287/S, www.worldbank.org accessed 7 February 2005.

———. 2005. *World development report 2005*. Oxford: Oxford University Press.

WTO. 2001. Declaration on the Trips Agreement and public health. WT/MIN(01)/DEC/2 20 November, www.wto.org accessed 6 August 2005.

———. 2003. Implementation of paragraph 6 of the Doha Declaration on the TRIPS Agreement and public health. WT/L/540 1 September, www.wto.org accessed 6 August 2005.

Yanco, J. 1996. Our Bodies, Ourselves in Beijing: breaking the silences. *Feminist Studies* 22(3):511–518.

Young, J. 1999. *The exclusive society.* London: Sage.

Zedner, L. 1995. Wayward sisters: the prison for women. In *The Oxford history of the prison* edited by N. Morris and D.J. Rothman, 329–361. New York: Oxford University.

Zibechi, R. 2005. New challenges for radical social movements. *NACLA Report on the Americas* March–April, 38(5):14.

Zola, I.K. 1989. Toward the necessary universalizing of a disability policy. *Milbank Quarterly* 67, Suppl. 2, Pt. 2: 401–428.

Zones, J.S. 1997. Beauty myths and realities and their impact on women's health. In *Women's health: complexities and differences* edited by S.B. Ruzek, V.L. Olesen, and A.E. Clarke, 249–275. Columbus: Ohio State University Press.

INDEX